APPROACHING
THE
'PAUSE

Candid conversations on the journey towards menopause

DR ROSIE ROSS ✳ **JOANNE VINES**

First published 2021 by Dr Rosie Ross and Joanne Vines

Produced by Indie Experts P/L, Australasia
indieexperts.com.au

Cover design by Daniela Catucci @ Catucci Design
Edited by Anne-Marie Tripp
Internal design by Indie Experts
Typeset by Post Pre-press Group, Brisbane

ISBN 978-0-6488209-3-2 (paperback)
ISBN 978-0-6488209-1-8 (epub)
ISBN 978-0-6488209-2-5 (kindle)

Disclaimer: The content of this book is for informational purposes only and is not intended to diagnose, treat, cure, or prevent any condition or disease. You understand that this book is not intended as a substitute for consultation with a licensed practitioner. Please consult with your own physician or healthcare specialist regarding the suggestions and recommendations made in this book. The use of this book implies your acceptance of this disclaimer.

This is our gift to you. A book to help you navigate your way through the 'pause with grace, dignity, knowledge and tears of joy!

It's time we all talked more about this transition into our third act in life. There is no time like the present, and so we invite you to spread the word so that from here forward none of our sisters need to battle through these transitional years alone in non-blissful ignorance.

Jo and Dr Rosie

Contents

Preface

Like you, I've gone through those uncertain times when life changed, and it was during my forties that older friends started to ask me about my journey towards menopause. As a GP who also came to that career choice later in life, having done nursing and naturopathy first, I had the advantage of having had many conversations with patients and with medical professionals I knew before 'the change' became front and centre of my own daily life.

Even then, as with pregnancy or raising children, I *thought* I knew what to expect from the wise council of elders and the books I'd read. The reality was somewhat different. As a GP, I have come to appreciate how each individual's menopausal journey is different. There are those who sail though their peri-menopausal transitioning years without (literally) breaking much of a sweat. And then there are many others who find themselves hot and sweaty and truly bothered as they realise their roaring forties were not at all how they imagined it might be. Many women during many consultations have brought their unique 'body of lived experience' and shared that they were not exactly sure what was going on with their bodies, and how they felt uncertain, unprepared and at times anxious because no one had really sat down and talked about the changes that can occur during this change-of-life stage.

Although we may never meet, I would like you to know that I wrote this book with you in mind. Whatever your personal journey towards 'the pause', I wanted to share with you the professional insights I've learned as a doctor who is truly passionate about women's wellbeing and health literacy, and – on a personal note – reassurance from a been-there-done-that, passionate menopausal woman that it is possible to not only survive but to thrive during these years. Having journeyed ahead of you, I have drawn you a map to help you prepare for your voyage as you navigate the next stage of your life. A chart of possible reefs and rocks. A plan on how to avoid icebergs that can sink your ship. Healthy lifestyle strategies you might consider steering your choices toward being your best version of yourself. And if you get the point of feeling washed out or washed up, calling on a helping hand from a medical or allied health professional.

All of us somewhere on the journey towards our exciting coming-of-age as wise sages and exotic wonderful wild women stepping into our power in our mid-later years. Our mission is to change the narrative surrounding how women navigate the years leading into menopause to enter what is potentially the most powerful phase of life.

With warmest wishes for your wellbeing,
Dr Rosie Ross
MBBS (Hons), BHSc (Nat Med) FRACGP

I was brought up in Melbourne, Victoria, in the 1970s with an Australian mother and a Maori father. In the Maori culture, the older you are the more respected you become. A *kuia* (female elder) is admired, respected and an integral part of the *whanau* (family). Younger generations are guided by her wisdom and knowledge of life experiences, especially when it comes to raising children, and her position as the matriarch is paramount to the *whanau*'s longevity. Her appearance is disregarded, and her ageing, curvaceous, fuller figure, greying wiry hair and wrinkles are honoured and add to her overall character.

What a shame that in some cultures, as women age, they are not treated with the level of respect they deserve and can feel irrelevant, worthless and past their use-by date. Individually, we need to appreciate our God-given natural beauty. We are not doing ourselves or each other any favours if we buy into this need for perfection.

I once looked forward to middle age. I was excited at the prospect of finally having time to myself, more sexy time with my husband and disposable income from being empty-nesters. I couldn't wait to embrace the flexibility of a lifestyle where I didn't always have to plan and cook evening meals or eat regularly if I didn't want to. Being able to trade the structured routines for opportunities to sleep, wake, nap, wash and eat whenever I wished was an exciting prospect. The grind of daily routine and the challenges of raising a family would be a thing of the past and life would be mine for the taking. How wrong I was: NO-ONE warned me that along with independence and financial freedom came perimenopause and ultimately menopause!

I don't ever remember my mother, aunties, grandmothers or mother-in-law sitting around over a cup of tea discussing perimenopause or menopause. We got the talk about periods and pregnancy when growing up and I thought we'd talked about everything else at school including sex, relationships, marriage and babies. But for some reason menopause was never a topic up for discussion. Why do we not speak openly about menopause and the transition that every woman will experience in her life? Why is it taboo in our homes and, overall, in society? Actually, I had never heard the word until I was well into my adult years. When I first learnt of the word 'perimenopause' from my GP, I hoped to breeze through this stage unscathed. However, nothing could prepare me for the unimaginable, radical transformation that would take place.

My body started changing before I realised and long before I thought I was of the appropriate age or stage of life to become 'all dried up and put out for pasture'. It's hard to deny notable hormonal changes, with irregular periods, mood swings, joint aches, insomnia, thinning hair, sleep deprivation, night sweats, hot flushes, itchiness, dryness, weight gain – especially around my middle – and my breasts and vagina have lost their plumpness. WOW! And this is only perimenopause – shoot me now! My eyebrow has dropped to my top lip, so I sport a monobrow and my crown jewel has now become a crown of thorns – ouch!

I get slapped in the face most days with body changes and every day heralds yet another surprise. When I woke to find a grey pubic hair, I screamed OMG! WTF! When I shared my disgust with a girlfriend, she said, "You're lucky; mine have nearly all dropped out." She was excited to learn she was now on trend with her unintentional Brazilian.

Another girlfriend shared her opinion on ageing, saying, "Just because your vaginal juices dry up doesn't mean the fluid in your brain dries too." She feels discarded, underrated, unappreciated and not valued as she ages. Her children jokingly tell her grandchildren not to take any notice of Grandma because she's just old and silly; Grandma is only 55. Grandma is exhausted both physically and emotionally from spending the last 30 years raising a family and putting everyone else first. She now looks at herself and feels disappointed that she did not take the time to care equally for herself and her family. She is paying the price with excess weight and lack of vitality. Her doctor has told her she may be prone to metabolic syndrome due to her high blood pressure. Finally, she now has time for herself but is expected to look after her grandchildren and ageing parents.

In our twenties, one of my girlfriends knew the importance of having a serious discussion with me about superannuation and retirement planning. If we'd known, maybe we could have spiced up the conversation by talking about how we could also plan for menopause! Now that it is here upon me, I wish I had been warned so that I could have prepared for the changes, physical and emotional, and made it a part of my life plan.

We need support to negotiate this emotional rollercoaster and advice on how to make it a smoother ride. It's hard not to feel ripped off, pissed off, out of control, and wanting to take a pause from life. Now, I am a woman possessed: I'm trying hard to find the humour in the madness by embracing my intuition and listening with sensitivity to what my body truly wants and needs. And wondering, am I part of a silent army of middle-aged women marching to the beat of the same drum?

I wrote this book with my friend, GP 'Dr Rosie', because we know there is much conversation to be had, and we don't all get to enjoy talking with our own mothers, aunties, sisters, friends or even our own daughters about what this transitional phase of life is all about. So, we decided to get together and explore the many weird and wonderful – yes, it's not all bad! – experiences common to us as we go through 'the change' and emerge into our 'Wonder Years'. If you are reading this book, you may have found yourself at the end of your youth and the beginning of your wonder years too. I hope that you will find support, comfort and knowledge to help you navigate these choppy, uncharted waters.

Always,
Joanne Vines

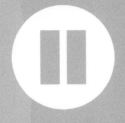

Chapter 1
PERIODS

It all started in the summer of '79!

I remember getting my period for the first time at 12. It was the summer of 1979.

I loved having a birthday in January as it was school holidays, so everyone was home and relaxed. We were allowed to have soft drink and lollies on the odd occasion, and we had lots of extended family coming and going. The weather was generally hot, it was daylight savings and we were all buzzing from having just celebrated the festive season. I remember it well: it was the summer of '79 and it's as clear in my memory today as if it was yesterday.

As teenagers, we had talked about getting our periods and were ever so embarrassed when we had to watch videos on the subject at school. 'The blossoming of a girl into a woman' was hard to take at age 12 in sex education class. Boys, periods and losing our virginities were topics of great discussions that fascinated me and I took a real interest.

When the big day finally arrived, it was not a joyful day to sing and rejoice, even though it had been sold to me that way. I was immediately upset and distressed, but luckily, I had an older sister who snapped into gear and knew the right process. She was so excited and clapped her hands then rushed from our joint bedroom to spread the word. Mum came straight in as if it was an emergency and said, "Well, it's time we had the talk!"

What talk? I thought. *Oh no, not that talk!*

"Let's talk about the birds and the bees," said Mum.

Quick to my feet and before Mum would say anything more embarrassing, I said, "Mum, you don't need to talk to me about the 'birds and the bees', I know everything – Tina told me!" Tina, who was 14, hadn't told me everything (which I would later discover), but I most definitely didn't want to hear 'the talk' from my Mum, on the MOST embarrassing day of my life. My brother Charles, also 12, had the task of rushing to Safeway to buy the pads. He was like Speedy Gonzales on his dragster bike and returned in a flash with a brown paper bag. How lovely and discreet buying pads was in those days!

And so it started, the 28-day cycle, in the summer of '79. Sounds like a song, but it was no hit in my world. My body felt every change, every month. I suffered PMT (premenstrual tension), known today as PMS (premenstrual syndrome). Painful cramping and uncontrollable bleeding plagued my period. My teenage years were a stressful, emotional time that only got worse as I aged. I was grateful to have 7 to 10 days per month where I would feel like myself, not bloated or worried that I would leak and have a big patch of blood on the back of my school tunic or work skirt.

As keen as we were to use tampons, being raised as a Catholic added moral complications. There was a myth that using tampons would rupture your hymen and technically you would no longer be a virgin. Yep, as crazy as it was, this was a big deal for Catholic girls.

Aunty Anne, Mum's sister, was her confidant and go-to. Mum could always rely on her younger sister in times of need. Aunty Anne only had toddlers at that point, but as she worked as a nurse she was up to date with life and all things period-related! As we were very active teenagers and involved in many different sports, adhesive pads weren't cutting it, especially in dancing. Our 'time of the month' was impacting our lifestyle and participation. To our surprise, one Saturday afternoon Aunty Anne arrived at our house with a mission: to teach us how to insert a tampon! The purpose was to have an understanding of our vagina and the direction in which we would need to insert the tampon, and this lesson allowed us to explore our vaginas in a safe and secure environment – and at least I found out that day that there is only one way in and out! We soon became professionals and the coolest girls at school. The safety of doubling up with both tampon and pad brought great relief until Mum decided there was another course of action to explore – the Pill!

Our Catholic upbringing also preached that the Pill was for 'racy non-Catholic good-time girls'. We thought that the Pill was used only for contraception and the girls who were taking it were wishing to have or having sex. There was a lot of ignorance around the Pill being a medical support for young women, so going on the Pill to regulate and control my period was an interesting and exciting concept. I was thrilled when my GP suggested the idea and couldn't wait to tell my closest girlfriends that Mum had willingly put me on the Pill. Mum insisted it wasn't a contraceptive pill and that it wouldn't stop me from getting pregnant, but considering I wasn't having sex, it would do the job! It was the summer of '81, I was 14 and on the Pill – so cool!

For the next few years, I tried and tested many different contraceptive pills, but nothing really helped control my periods. I would have the odd good month where I'd manage to breeze through with little pain or shame, although my bed linen always revealed the true story – which reminds me of how non-discreet it must have been using sanitary towels before disposable sanitary items were available. So, you could imagine my relief the day my period stopped for the first time since it had begun; I was 16, it was the summer of '83.

Our GP was Mum's friend and she had decided to trial me on a 'medical curette' as I had become anaemic and unwell because my periods were so heavy. This was administered by a course of tablets that would allow the uterine lining to pass on its own accord – a much less invasive procedure than surgery. I was several months into the trial when I told my mum that I was concerned that I hadn't had a period for months. Mum called her GP friend, who dropped by on her way home. Although she had planned to examine me, instead she caught up with my mum over a drink all whilst I waited for a diagnosis. As she was walking out the door to leave, I prompted Mum to share my concerns about not passing the 'uterine lining'. She reassured Mum and me that my body would take its natural course when ready. The question of being sexually active wasn't raised and I was enjoying feeling fabulous for the first time in my life. You could imagine everyone's surprise when I discovered two weeks later that I was 25 weeks pregnant – and that's another story and book! 'Thou shalt not have sex before marriage.' Whoops!

Nevertheless, while my periods always caused havoc, they never disappointed, turning up right on time every 28 days. But now, they are irregular, which is frustrating to say the least. Holidays and sexy times away have always been planned around my cycle, but now I can't be guaranteed if and when they might show up unexpectedly. You'd think I'd be embracing this time, excited with the knowledge that I'm nearing the end of the dreaded years. Soon, free to wear white jeans! I guess that's why so many middle-aged women wear white pedal pushers – because they can!

I can't believe that there's a part of me that's missing my 'monthlies'. Mourning the loss of a familiar friend, a tumultuous relationship that once ruled my life. There's a sense of sadness, knowing that my baby-breeding days are done (of course they were years ago), but that's not the point. Contraception will be a thing of the past; the ebb and flow of the moon that once signalled to my body that it was time, and the build-up of stress and tension that would naturally release on impact will be no longer.

The summer of 2020 has marked another milestone: my dreaded period seems to have stopped for the last five months. And just when I should be celebrating, I now can't sleep and my body's on fire – GREAT!

Dear Dr Rosie,

My monthly cycles have been all over the place recently, and five months ago they stopped entirely. Sometimes I feel like I am on fire with hot flushes and I'm having trouble sleeping. What the hell! Have I suddenly hit menopause? I hope you don't mind but I have a few questions I need answered:

- What is menopause and why does it happen?
- When do I know that I'm officially in menopause?
- Are there any clues when my final menstrual period may occur?
- At what age does menopause occur?
- What is perimenopause and how long will it last?

Thanks,
Jo

Let's talk about periods

Hi Jo,

Thank you for your letter, I was pleased to hear from you. I'll get straight down to answering your questions about your erratic menstrual cycles, not having a period for the past few months, and the fact that you have started having hot flushes and are wondering whether or not you are in menopause. I can understand it can be very confusing; I find that many of the women I speak with tend to think that hot flushes must automatically mean they are in menopause. However, as we delve into this letter, we are going find that that is not necessarily the case. To start with, let me be clear, Jo: if you're still having a menstrual cycle, no matter how irregular that menstrual cycle is, you are not yet menopausal.

What is menopause and why does it happen?

Based on the biology of sex hormones, a woman's life is divided into different stages: infancy and childhood, puberty, reproductive, perimenopause, menopause and postmenopause. The natural fertile reproductive years are bounded by menarche (our first menstrual period) and menopause (12 months after the final menstrual period). The transition phase to the time of finally crossing the menopause line is called perimenopause, which means 'the time around menopause', and the time after crossing that menopause line is called postmenopause, which is the rest of your life.

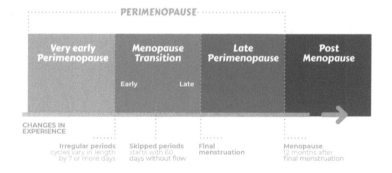

Once upon an ovary

A woman's reproductive stage of life starts with menarche and it involves ovaries, eggs and hormones. We have two ovaries. Our eggs are each cradled within follicles in the ovaries. The follicles also make hormones such as oestrogen and progesterone. The ovary's functioning capacity decreases with age. Over the course of a woman's lifetime, the number of eggs and follicles also declines.

Did you know that we have the greatest number of eggs, around six to seven million, whilst we are still within our mother's womb? If you look at the diagram on the next page, you will see that at birth, a woman has between one and two million eggs in her ovaries. A few at a time, these eggs are awoken at puberty by surges of two hormones that are made in the brain, follicle-stimulating hormone and luteinising hormone. At the time of puberty there are around 400,000 eggs left; however, only 10 per cent of these eggs will mature and somewhere between 300 to 400 eggs will be released during a woman's reproductive lifetime. As the number of follicles and eggs continues to decline during the midlife, hormones start to fluctuate and the menstrual bleeding pattern starts to change during perimenopause. By the time we reach natural menopause, there are about 1000 of our original eggs left.

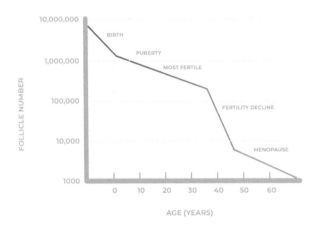

Menopause occurs when the number of ovarian follicles has declined to a point where there are no longer enough follicles to produce sufficient ovarian oestrogen hormones that stimulate the release of eggs and therefore menstrual cycles stop permanently. Although the decline in both follicles and eggs is a predictable trend, the release of hormonal ovarian oestrogen during the perimenopausal transition may be much more erratic and unpredictable[1]. Some months a small amount of oestrogen is released and other times there is a large amount of oestrogen released. What that means is that some months an egg is released and other months no egg is released. It is the decline in the number of follicles and changes in levels of hormones made by the follicles that are responsible for many of the symptoms a woman may experience during the perimenopausal and menopausal phase of her life.

We often hear that the interplay of our sex hormones is like a symphony played in a harmony of regular, well-orchestrated cycles. Although oestrogen and progesterone made in our ovaries are probably the sex hormones we are most familiar with, there are other hormones involved like follicle-stimulating hormone and luteinising hormone which are made in our brains.

As the hormonal 'orchestra' 'tunes up' during the puberty years, the irregular, erratic hormonal ups and downs can result in an ovary sometimes releasing an egg (ovulatory cycle) and other times not releasing an egg (anovulatory cycle). These erratic ovulation patterns can be reflected in erratic menstrual cycles and emotional turbulence with mood swings.

Over time, adolescents mature into adulthood, and the adult reproductive years tend to be calmer with oestrogen, progesterone and other sex hormones rising and falling in a regular pattern.

During the reproductive phase, hormones tend to rise and fall in a fairly predictable pattern over the length of a normal menstrual cycle. The menstrual cycle starts at day one of our period and ends on the day before your next menstrual bleed. Cycle length is highly variable and on average lasts anywhere from 21 to 35 days[2]. Whilst most charts and diagrams show the 28-day cycle, in fact only about 15 per cent of women have 28-day cycles[3].

Eventually, more changes take place and adults' peak reproductive years transition into the perimenopause phase where oestrogen and progesterone level patterns become disrupted. Ovaries start to release eggs erratically again, which in turn makes menstrual cycles erratic in the lead up to when ovaries no longer release eggs at all. These changes are illustrated in the diagram below.

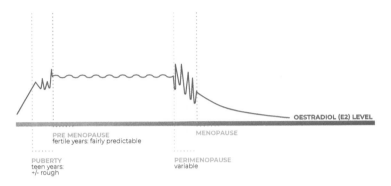

It might be useful at this point to explain a bit more about oestrogen and what it does.

The oestrogen family

Oestrogen is a family of three different hormones that act in a similar way.

- Oestrone (E1). This is a weaker type of oestrogen produced in the ovaries, fat cells and adrenal glands. This is the main type of oestrogen produced after a woman moves into menopause.
- Oestradiol (E2). Also called 17 beta-estradiol, this is the strongest type of oestrogen and is mainly produced in the ovaries. While oestradiol has many functions, its main job is to mature, regulate and maintain the female reproductive system. It is responsible for the development of female secondary sexual characteristics such as breasts, widening hips, and fat distribution, the development of internal sex organs, as well as the maturation and release of eggs during

ovulation. Oestradiol levels vary throughout the menstrual cycle, increasing to their highest levels at ovulation and dropping to their lowest at menstruation. Oestradiol binds to our oestrogen receptors the most strongly and is therefore most potent. In terms of potency, oestradiol is 10 times stronger than oestrone (E1) and 100 times more potent than oestriol (E3). Oestradiol production decreases as a woman ages, with the largest drop occurring during menopause. This decrease, however, is not gradual, and oestradiol production can fluctuate wildly during perimenopause.

* Oestriol (E3). Another weaker type of oestrogen, oestriol is mainly produced by the placenta during pregnancy. Oestriol levels increase throughout a pregnancy, and are at their highest levels just before birth.

When oestradiol levels swing up to a high level, we may experience symptoms of breast tenderness and swelling. One lady told me that sometimes her breasts "blew up like balloons" and she used a bra three times bigger than her regular bras for just those seven to ten days of the month before her period was due. Fluid retention can also cause any rings we wear on our fingers to feel tighter. Other signs of higher oestradiol levels during the cycle can include bloating, premenstrual syndrome (PMS), headaches, heavy menstrual flooding and mood swings. When oestradiol levels drop to their lowest point during menstruation, we tend to feel symptoms that we might associate with menopause such as hot flushes, night sweats and a difficulty to concentrate. As your hormones are swinging up and down erratically, is it any wonder that you may sometimes feel as though you have premenstrual syndrome 24/7?

Highs and lows of the erratic oestradiol see-saw of perimenopause

HIGHS AND LOWS OF THE ERRATIC OESTRADIOL SEE-SAW OF PERIMENOPAUSE

HIGH OESTROGEN SYMPTOMS
Breast tenderness and swelling
Bloating
Fluid retention
PMS
Mood swings
Headaches

LOW OESTROGEN SYMPTOMS
Hot flashes
Irregular periods
Painful intercourse
Difficulty concentrating
More frequent urinary tract infections
Fatigue

It is not uncommon for women who are experiencing the hormonal ups and downs of perimenopause to comment that it feels like they are revisiting puberty. But this time around, it can feel like puberty on steroids. The main difference this time around is that the social context has changed and there may be an overlay of work-life balance pressures, issues with work commitments, relationship concerns, ageing parents or their own health problems. For some, trying to find balance amidst these multiple stressors is further compounded by the challenge of limited financial resources.

When do I know that I am officially in menopause?

When your final menstrual period is followed by 12 months of no further menstrual cycles and therefore your periods have stopped permanently, then and only then may you consider that you have officially arrived at a natural menopause. It can be a bit tricky to know at the time if 'this is it', your last ever menstrual period, because you will not know whether 'that was it' until at least 12 months after the fact. If your last menstrual period was only five months ago, you cannot be certain that you have entered menopause yet.

Are there any clues when my final menstrual period may occur?

I agree that it would be helpful to have an idea about when our final menstrual period might occur. A common scenario for women in the lead up to their final menstrual period is to have no period for two months, then normal cycles with a menstrual flow for the next three months, followed by minimal spotting (which may look more like a smear), and then nothing for 10 months. You think you're almost there and then *bang!*, another bleed. A 52-year-old woman shared that after no sign of her cycle for 11 months and two days, she gathered up her pads and tampons and was about to bid them a ceremonial farewell when ... it happened. Apparently, there was a lot of weeping, wailing and wild words, with a few things thrown. Thankfully, they were all soft objects.

The perimenopause transition is divided into two parts, an early and a late stage. In the early stage of the perimenopausal transition, menstrual cycles tend to be regular with a few interruptions; however, one of the signposts of this transition is a change in cycle length of seven or more days for at least three consecutive menstrual cycles[4]. What that means is that, on one hand, the time between menstrual cycles may get shorter by at least seven days and periods start to arrive closer together, while on the other hand, they might stretch out by at least seven days so that consecutive cycles become fewer and further apart. In the late stage, anywhere from one to three years before the final menstrual period, menstrual cycles start to stretch out to more than 60 days apart.

However, remember that individual variability? Not all women will transition this way. You may be comforted to know that 15 to 25 per cent of women will experience no change or only minimal changes in their menstrual cycles from their regular menstrual cycle rhythm prior to their final menstrual period, which only goes to underline that every woman is progressing on her individual journey. Some women may have regular cycles and then one day they miss their menstrual period ... and that is the end of that.

At what age does menopause occur?

A natural menopause occurs anywhere between 45 and 55 years of age, and on average, a Western woman crosses the natural menopause line at 51.4 years. However, every woman is different and a lot of variability is still possible, so it can happen anywhere between the ages of 40 and 58 years. The median age when a woman starts perimenopause is 47.5 years[5].

There are some women who may experience menopause at an earlier age, between 41 and 45 years. This is called an **early menopause**. If a woman's mother or sister(s) have had an early menopause, then there is a greater possibility that this will be her experience too. An early menopause can happen if a woman has a hysterectomy, which includes the surgical removal of ovaries. Women undergoing various cancer treatments, such as chemotherapy or radiotherapy to their pelvic area, will experience menopause at the time of having those treatments. Some autoimmune conditions and genetic conditions can also lead to an early or premature menopause. When we talk about **premature menopause**, we are talking about this event occurring before the age of 40.

How long will this perimenopause transition stage last?

Well, it depends. It depends because each and every one of us is different and our genetic inheritance, ethnicity, culture and personal behaviours can have an influence. Just as there are many different women, there are many variations on the length of time of a 'normal', natural transition phase. Some women pass through that transition phase in as little as two years whilst others may take six to eight years[6]. On average, the perimenopausal transition phase takes four to five years. However, if you are a smoker, you may cross the menopause line one to two years earlier[7].

Remembering that the perimenopause transition is a natural change that occurs in a woman's life, you may wonder if there are occasions when it would be advisable to see your doctor. If you are having menstrual bleeds that are heavier than usual, menstrual periods that occur more frequently than every three weeks, or bleeding that is lasting longer than three weeks or bleeding in between your cycles, or if you have passed into menopause (no cycles for 12 months) and then you start to bleed again or bleed after having intercourse, it would be wise to book an appointment with your health professional. I know you, Jo, have not reached this stage yet, however, if you or any woman you know has passed into menopause (no cycles for 12 months) and then you start to bleed again or bleed after having intercourse, this is what is called a 'red flag' (no pun intended). A red flag is an indicator there may be a serious underlying condition that needs further investigation and definitely when you need to make a doctor's appointment quick smart.

I realise that I have been talking about a woman who is transitioning into a natural menopause and not mentioned a woman who has had a surgical or chemical intervention. In the case of a woman who has had a hysterectomy or endometrial ablation, or her pelvis has been irradiated, tracking cycles can be a little tricky without menstrual blood-flow patterns or if she is under the age of 45 and experiencing symptoms that may suggest she is actually menopausal. In these cases, there is a blood test that can be arranged by a doctor to check your level of follicle-stimulating hormone (FSH). The test is taken as a baseline and repeated at a 6-week interval. If the FSH level is raised above the normal level, it is suggestive of menopause. At that time, it's best to book in for a 'Well Woman' health check to discuss her results because hormone deficiencies can impact both short- and long-term health.

Now getting back to you Jo, and your natural perimenopausal transition. The last thing I shall say here, is that although you have no control over the passage of time and the fact that your body is changing, what you *can* choose is to master your midlife and make your perimenopausal years *positively life changing*. With recent advances in evidence-based information it is possible to embrace change, make lifestyle choices that sustain your self-care, put your hand up and access help from a range of health professionals if you need it and get ready to step over the threshold of menopause into the next powerful stage of your life as a healthy, well-thy and wise woman.

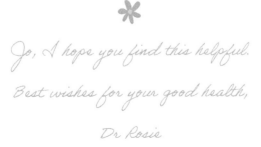

Jo, I hope you find this helpful.

Best wishes for your good health,

Dr Rosie

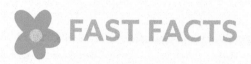 # FAST FACTS

When do I know that I'm officially in menopause?

When your final menstrual period is followed by 12 months of no further menstrual cycles and therefore your periods have stopped permanently, then and only then may you consider that you have officially arrived at a natural menopause.

At what age does menopause occur?

Menopause usually occurs between the ages of 45 and 55. In Australia, the average age is 51.4 years.

Early menopause is considered to occur between the ages of 41 and 45.

Menopause that occurs before the age of 40 is considered **premature**.

Are there any clues when my final menstrual period may occur?

In the early stages of the perimenopausal transition, menstrual cycles tend to be regular, but one of the signposts that this transition has started is a change in cycle length: time between menstrual cycles may get shorter and periods may start arriving closer together, or time between cycles may get longer and periods arrive further apart. This may give you an indication that your final period is on its way. Some women, however, experience no change, or minimal changes, in their menstrual cycle in the lead up to their final period.

What is this thing I hear called perimenopause and is this it? And how long will it last?

The transition phase leading up to finally crossing the menopause line is called perimenopause (meaning 'around the menopause'). Some women pass through this transition phase in as little as two years whilst others may take six to eight years. On average, the perimenopausal phase takes four to five years.

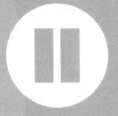

Chapter 2
CONTRACEPTION

Safety in numbers!

I'm glad that I've finally found something positive in sliding down the dry, no longer slippery slope into menopause: not having to worry about contraception – yippee!

There were many years of heartache, worrying about taking the Pill. Where was a safe place I could leave it so that I'd remember to take it at the same time each day? On my bedside so it was the first thing I'd see in the morning, next to my toothbrush in the bathroom vanity unit as I'd never leave home before brushing my teeth, in the teabag canister as I'd always need a cup of tea before I faced the day, in the fridge next to the milk, just in case I was having a bad morning and missed it with the teabags, and if all else failed, in my running shoes, as exercise is a morning ritual and I was bound to find it before I shoved my foot in my shoe. I felt safer and more at ease if I'd covered all bases. Let's face it, I was an expert at slipping up, so I became paranoid about another unplanned pregnancy.

It didn't matter how creative or ridiculous my prompts were, there was always a day or two that I missed while taking the Pill, and then it was on – or, actually, it was off! No sex in our household for two weeks! The red flag would also go up after a bout of vomiting or diarrhoea and the exclusion zone would be in place again.

My husband had his own agenda and interests at heart and therefore could provide a condom in a blink of the eye just in case I weakened. He had wet checks, frangers, condoms and rubbers all over the house, and in the car! All types of textures, colours, flavours and sizes.

He was as innovative about hiding these as I was about putting my Pills in places to remind me to take them, so he probably also hid one in his shoe. No surprise, he became very persistent at reminding me nearly every day of our married life for the first 10 years.

"Have you taken your pill?" was a regular question over morning coffee.

"Yes, darling," was music to his ears; this sexy talk always ensured his day started with a big smile.

And then came the smartphone.

The smartphone has been revolutionary in taking the stress out of taking the Pill. Reminding us what we're doing, where we're going, at what time, with whom, how many times and for what reason. Recently I was on a business trip with a team member and we shared an apartment. I hadn't realised until she brought it to my attention that I have many daily, weekly, and annual reminders: wake up, go to bed, take morning vitamins, take evening magnesium, do payroll, collect grandchildren, call bookkeeper, call accountant, check blood pressure, get a massage, watch favourite TV programs – and that's just Fridays! There are no excuses for missing anything in today's world.

How easy life would have been in the 'good old days' if I had had an iPhone. It would have saved me from having to come up with ridiculous places to stash the Pill and it would have given my husband peace of mind – and a lot more sex!

Being Catholic also meant that abortion wasn't an option and I would go to hell for even considering such a thing, so I considered every other precaution. "Better to be safe than sorry," was my catchcry, although now that I reflect on it, it reminds me how uptight, crazy, regimented, paranoid and over-the-top I became about taking one tiny little white pill. How an incy-wincy tablet would be the catalyst for how the rest of my life would play out. Nevertheless, the ramifications of not taking the pill were enormous.

Natural planning (AKA the 'rhythm method'), where you tracked your cycle on a calendar to predict your time of ovulation and abstained from sex on your fertile days, felt like playing Russian Roulette. Although perfect for those who were risk takers and liked to gamble, it was definitely not an option for me!

I considered a hysterectomy after having my children but decided it was a little extreme. It was one way of taking care of contraception indefinitely, but also meant I might slip into early menopause, a chance I wasn't prepared to take at 28.

Later, I was introduced to the Mirena IUD. What an amazing discovery. Just like the iPhone, it revolutionised contraception in our household. Our sex life was finally no longer dependent on reminders, and stress was reserved for other things. Set a reminder in your diary five years from now to have it replaced.

Even when my husband had a vasectomy, I opted for contraception for a further six months until I could be guaranteed I was safe.

For some of my girlfriends, their periods come and go so contraception has now become a thing of the past and they are embracing being off the Pill after 30-plus years. Others are enjoying not having the irritation and inflammation of regular condom use. Contraception is no longer at the forefront of their minds and they're loving the satisfaction of being promiscuous and carefree.

Dear Dr Rosie,

- When is it safe to stop using contraception?
- If I still need contraception, what are my options?
- What is a change-of-life baby?

Thanks,
Jo

Let's talk about contraception

Hi Jo,

Good to hear from you, but first things first. If you are still having menstrual periods, no matter how irregular they are, if you are sexually active, it is *really* important to ensure you protect yourself and have some reliable form of contraception in place. Your husband has had a vasectomy, so that is contraception sorted for you (as long as you are monogamous). However, in case some of your friends are wondering aloud, you might like to share what follows with them.

Whilst we tend to notice the variability in our menstrual cycles, what we may not realise is that the change in our menstrual cycle pattern mirrors the variability in the release of an egg from our ovaries. Some months an egg will be released, but over time as we approach menopause, there will be more and more months when no egg is released. Although we know that perimenopause is a time when fertility potential has decreased, to have sex without the protection of a reliable form of contraception can be a gamble.

When is it safe to stop using contraception?

You wondered how long a woman is advised to use contraception. If a woman is not yet 50 and has had her final menstrual period before she turned 50, then it is recommended to continue using contraceptive measures for two years after that final menstrual period. If a woman has had her final menstrual period after turning 50 years old, then it is recommended to use contraception for another 12 months. Of course, there are exceptions here. If you are not sexually active, have a same-sex partner, have had a hysterectomy or a tubal ligation, or your partner has had a vasectomy, then the need for contraception to prevent pregnancy is not an issue. If you do require protection against sexually transmitted infections, then condoms are a good option to use or to continue using.

If I still need contraception, what are my options?

What are your options for contraception during the lead-up time to menopause? Briefly, there are non-hormonal and hormonal options. Non-hormonal options include abstinence, fertility awareness methods (FAMs), barrier methods such as condoms, diaphragms, copper intrauterine devices (IUDs), and permanent methods such as surgical sterilisation by having a tubal ligation, or your partner may have a vasectomy. Condoms provide an additional benefit of protection from sexually transmitted infections (STIs) – especially for people who are not in monogamous relationships – and with consistent use, they are a worthwhile consideration – although there have been reports of reduced sensitivity which may affect sexual pleasure, and some people have an allergy or sensitivity to latex. Condoms do come in a latex-free option, though. A copper IUD lasts five to ten years depending on the type; however, this form of contraception may be associated with heavier, more painful periods.

Hormonal options most suitable for women in perimenopause are the oral contraceptive pill and a progestogen-only intrauterine device (IUD) called Mirena in Australia. The combined oral contraceptive pill contains both oestrogen and progestogen. In addition to the contraceptive protection it provides, many women experience its benefit of regulating their previously erratic menstrual cycles, reducing flushes and improving bone health. However, the oestrogen component of the combined pill is not suitable for every woman, especially if she is over 50, a smoker, has high blood pressure, Type 2 diabetes or is of an unhealthy weight.

If a contraceptive slip-up does occur, emergency contraception ('the morning-after pill') is available to take after unprotected sex and can be bought over the counter from a pharmacy without a prescription. The name is a misnomer however, as it can be taken up to 72 hours (three days) after unprotected sex. In Australia, there is another emergency contraceptive pill that requires a prescription from your doctor and can be taken up to 120 hours (five days) after unprotected sex or a condom accident. However, neither of these are recommended as a routine form of contraception.

What is a change-of-life baby?

We know that fertility declines with age. A woman's fertility begins to decline in her late twenties and has further decreased by her late thirties. Although we know that fertility significantly declines from the age of 40, and continues to decline after the age of 50, the risk of conceiving is low but it is definitely NOT ZERO. Did you know that the oldest natural birth known was to a lady in the UK who had a baby at the age of 59 after conceiving naturally?

Jo, I hope you find this helpful.

Best wishes for your good health,

Dr Rosie

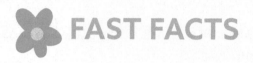 **FAST FACTS**

What are my contraception options?

There are non-hormonal and hormonal options. Non-hormonal options include abstinence, barrier methods such as condoms or diaphragms, copper intrauterine devices (IUDs) and permanent methods such as surgical sterilisation by having a tubal ligation, or your partner may have a vasectomy. Hormonal options include a combined (oestrogen and progestogen) oral contraceptive pill or a progestogen-only device such as a Mirena IUD. Make an appointment with your doctor to discuss your contraceptive preferences and the options that would best suit you.

When is it safe to stop using contraception?

If a woman is still having a menstrual cycle, no matter how erratic, she is considered perimenopausal because she has not crossed the menopause line. Although her risk of conceiving is low, her risk is NOT ZERO and a reliable form of contraception is advised. Remember, menopause is considered as twelve months after the final menstrual period.

Generally, if you have had your final menstrual period before the age of 50, then it is recommended to continue using contraceptive measures for two years after that final menstrual period. If you had your final menstrual period after turning 50, then it is recommended to use contraception for another twelve months.

What is a change-of-life baby?

Whilst fertility significantly declines around the age of 40, there is still a risk of conceiving. There is a low – but not zero – risk of conception if you engage in unprotected sex. The oldest known woman to give birth after conceiving naturally was 59 years old, in the UK.

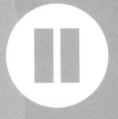

Chapter 3
WEIGHT GAIN

Middle-tyre disease

Today I woke to find a spare tyre around my middle! I'm sure it wasn't there yesterday or the day before ... well, maybe it was, maybe just a little, but today it is on show for all to see!

How did my once cute love handles become back fat and miraculously overnight turn into front fat? I've always embraced my voluptuous curves – well, I really didn't have a choice, but this is something new and totally on a different level. My middle is getting thicker and thicker ... apple-like ... maybe even *pregnant-like*! I can't help but notice that my friends' hourglasses have become apples too.

Have they caught what I've got – the middle-tyre disease?

This is truly an epidemic! A disease affecting most of my middle-age girlfriends, their friends and sisters. Many of them come from different cultures and backgrounds, but their stories are similar to mine. They are living the same way, doing the same things; we haven't changed our lifestyles, but our bodies are changing right before our eyes.

Is this a time to panic? Should we be taking this seriously and, hitting the gym more, saying no-no to anything that even resembles a carbohydrate – not even a smell, let alone a taste? Do we need to farewell our friend sugar; and what about champagne and the daily glass of wine? Some would prefer to sacrifice a child rather than give up alcohol!

What happened to excess weight being distributed on our bums and thighs? It could make one feel a little sensual and attractive at times, and a delight for many of our partners. But that brings me to that last bastion of womanhood – the dreaded control brief, tummy-control wear. For years, we managed to avoid the back corner of the lingerie stores, but now I see myself heading straight past the skimpy, lacy, strappy colourful stuff and am forced to face reality!

Did you know there's a control garment for every part of a woman's body, from her neck down to her knee, including a G-string? I know this because I have them all, including the boy leg, the full brief, the half brief, the skirt, the full dress, the under-the-bust-to-knee, and even the *under-the-bust-over-the-shoulder-to-knee*, in two colours: beige and black.

I remember as a young girl assisting my mother into what she referred to as her 'roll-ons'. My mother-in-law from the country calls them 'step-ins' but, honestly, these garments are like straightjackets – well, what I imagine one would feel like. I have no idea who came up with that ridiculous name for it, but at the end of the day they are all about sucking it in, pushing it up and keeping it there!

There was certainly no 'stepping-in' going on in our household when the control garment was required. Complete with beehive and false eyelashes, our mum would summon my sister Tina and me to her bedroom for the dressing to commence. We were well equipped and experienced for the task that could not be done single-handedly. Tina would position herself in front of Mum and I would be at the rear. On the count of three, we would hold our breath and heave. There would be some stops and starts along the way, and rarely did our first attempt to minimise Mum go to plan. But we never gave up until all of Mum's bits and pieces were pushed and squeezed and tucked in like a sausage. It was a satisfying job when completed and always left us breathless!

I called it shape-wear in my thirties, which was used to achieve no undie line; control-wear in my forties to pull in a few extra bumps I had acquired over the previous decade; and now, in my fifties, it's miracle-wear. Having worn these elasticised straitjackets for the past 20 years, I now pray for a miracle that they will fit and perform the magic they claim to.

However, the miracle-wear has its own issue with distributing the signs of the middle-tyre disease showing up unannounced in all kinds of places – under my arms, under my bust, on my back, under my neck, on my chin, on my thighs: there's frankly nowhere to hide. Gone are the days of wearing a belt. Bending over to tie up my shoelaces cuts off my windpipe, and sucking in my stomach doesn't feel natural anymore.

If you haven't discovered the polo shirt, now is the time. Men's polos are a little – actually, a lot – more comfortable than the ladies' polos. The right-sized polo provides the 'square drop' look from the top with no contact to any part of the upper body; a perfect staple item for the wardrobe. I am happy to age gracefully but preferably with some kind of a waistline.

Dear Dr Rosie,

- Why do so many midlife women gain weight?
- Why is gaining weight around my middle a problem?
- How can I know if I am an unhealthy weight?
- How can I know if I have metabolic syndrome?
- What can I do to reduce my middle tyre?

Thanks,
Jo

Let's talk about weight gain

Hi Jo,

I'm hearing your frustration with perimenopausal weight gain and a widening waistline because this happens to be a very common problem for women in their middle years. I often hear ladies lament, "I haven't changed what I'm eating, and I haven't done anything differently with my exercise routine, but all of a sudden, I have piled on five, ten, maybe more kilos. I promise you, I'm eating like a sparrow." And I believe them.

Why do so many midlife women gain weight?

It is an often-mistaken belief that weight gain is simply due to a lack of willpower; however, this is not the case. There are several different reasons for midlife weight gain that have little to do with willpower, such as increasing age, genetics, the influence of our environment that switches on or switches off our genes (epigenetics), hormones, sleep deprivation, lack of physical activity, gut microbiota, inflammation, and certain medications.

Ageing

It seems that women around midlife have a tendency to put on weight[1]. The Australian Longitudinal Study on Women's Health (2017)[2] followed the health of over 13,000 Australian women aged 45–50 years over a 20-year period and found that on average, the women participating in this study gained around five kilos in weight. On top of that, the US-based Study of Women's Health Across the Nation (SWAN)[3] discovered that over a three-year period, on average, the women in the study gained 2.1 kg in weight and 2.2 cm on their waist measurement. Similar weight gain findings were reported in a couple of other studies and it was concluded that women in their forties and early fifties, on average, gain 0.7 kg (1.5 lb) per year. According to these studies, ageing has an impact on weight gain, but why might that be?

As we age, our body composition changes, in that we tend to put on fat and lose lean muscle mass[4]. And that change in body composition can happen even if the numbers on bathroom scales tell us that our weight has stayed the same[5].

Why is body composition and the ratio of fat to lean muscle important? The number of calories we burn at rest is linked to our body composition, and specifically, the amount of lean muscle mass we have. Now, with less lean muscle mass, the number of calories that the body burns at rest (basal metabolic rate) starts to decrease by one to two per cent every 10 years after we turn 20. When we talk about basal metabolic rate, we mean the amount of energy the body needs for basic functioning: keeping the heart beating, breathing, thinking, digesting food and moving muscles. Perhaps by now you understand that if you eat the same amount of food as you always have (energy in), but your body now has less lean muscle to burn calories at rest and therefore a lower metabolic rate (energy out), you are going to put on weight.

Genetics

Genetics influence a wide range of our physical traits – our eye colour, whether or not our hair is curly or straight, how tall we are. They also influence our body shape and size, our metabolic rate and where we have a tendency to put on weight. If our parents and close family members have a tendency to put on weight easily, then there is a greater likelihood that we will too; but it does not mean this is inevitable. Dr. Judith Stern, Professor of Nutrition and Internal Medicine at the University of California is oft quoted as saying, "Genetics load the gun, but environment pulls the trigger," which means that although genetics have an influence on weight, our environment and lifestyle can have a positive or negative impact at the level of our genes. What that means is that the lifestyle choices we make can have a positive impact on managing our weight.

Hormones

Although ageing can result in less lean muscle tissue and contribute to weight gain, *where* that fat tends to be laid down in the body is due to genetic predisposition and the changes in levels of sex hormones during perimenopause. Do you remember your pre-puberty years when your body was straight up and down, and you looked forward to having boobs? When oestrogen kicks in at puberty, subcutaneous fat is laid down on the breasts, hips, buttocks and thighs, giving many young women a more curvaceous shape. In addition to oestrogen, several other hormones also influence our weight, including insulin, leptin, ghrelin (the hunger hormone), and GLP-1 – but they are well beyond the scope of this letter.

Subcutaneous (*sub* meaning under and *cutaneous* meaning skin) fat is the pinchable just-under-the-skin muffin-top fat or the dimpling-wobbly-cellulite fat that shows up on thighs or buttocks and has been the bane of many a woman's life. Your genetic lottery will influence whether you have an hourglass, pear, or rectangular silhouette. During perimenopause, the ovarian production of oestrogen shifts down a gear and with it there is a redistribution of fat to the abdomen, which gives women a widening waistline and more of an apple-shaped appearance[6]. Even women who weigh the same as they have in previous years and can maintain their relatively shapely arms and legs may discover that their waist gets thicker and they develop a little pot belly[7].

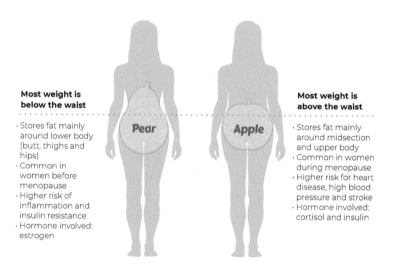

Most weight is below the waist

· Stores fat mainly around lower body (butt, thighs and hips)
· Common in women before menopause
· Higher risk of inflammation and insulin resistance
· Hormone involved: estrogen

Pear

Apple

Most weight is above the waist

· Stores fat mainly around midsection and upper body
· Common in women during menopause
· Higher risk for heart disease, high blood pressure and stroke
· Hormone involved: cortisol and insulin

But why, you might ask, does gaining weight really matter? I am mindful that weight and weight gain is a sensitive issue so please understand that any comments are not about body shaming; they are motivated by a 'keeping you healthy' perspective. From a health point of view, there is a large body of scientific evidence to suggest that being of an unhealthy weight[8] can increase our likelihood of developing a number of chronic medical conditions down the track, as you can see in my drawing below. Of particular concern is excess weight gain around the middle, called abdominal obesity.

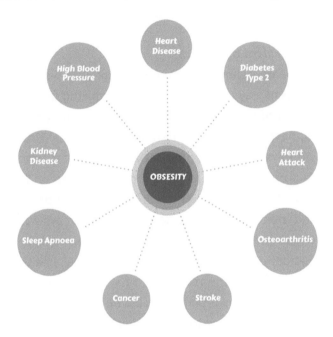

Why is gaining weight around my middle a problem?

Well, apart from not being able to zip up your favourite skinny jeans, it seems that as our waist measurement increases, so too do our health risks. A larger waist measurement associated with abdominal obesity is like a warning signpost of possible danger ahead in the form of insulin resistance[9], Type 2 diabetes[10] and heart disease[11].

You see, the belly fat involved in abdominal obesity may be made up of two different types of fat. There is the subcutaneous fat we already know about. And then there is the visceral fat. Visceral fat lies deeper inside and in normal amounts is helpful as it wraps around our liver, heart, kidneys, gallbladder and pancreas to cushion and protect them. Visceral fat becomes dangerous when there is too much of it and it shows up as belly fat and a thickened waistline.

Why is visceral fat a problem?

For many years, scientists thought that fat cells were simply a very efficient way to store extra calories during times when food was plentiful, and we could carry around our own energy supply to have on hand for when food was scarce. However, when we have excess visceral fat stores, this fat functions like a factory, actively churning out hormones and body chemicals – like leptin, adiponectin, tumour necrosis factor alpha, and Interleukin 6 to name a few[12] – that mess with our appetite and energy balance, as well as increasing low-level inflammation, all of which affect our physical health and mental wellbeing. Some researchers have called this excess visceral fat 'sick fat' as it plays havoc with our metabolic rate and results in a tendency to put on weight more easily, especially around the middle. An unhealthy amount of visceral fat in the abdomen has been linked with abnormal cholesterol levels, such as increased total cholesterol, LDL (bad) cholesterol and triglycerides, while at the same time lowering our HDL (good) cholesterol and increasing the risk of developing insulin resistance and diabetes type 2.

Insulin resistance occurs when the body does not respond to the normal effects of the hormone insulin. The pancreas makes insulin in response to eating carbohydrates (which our body breaks down into simple sugars like glucose) and, to a lesser extent, proteins. Insulin is like a key that unlocks the door to our muscle, liver and fat cells and helps glucose move out of our blood stream and into those cells where it can be used as fuel, or the glucose can be stored as glycogen in our muscles and liver cells. Insulin is also involved in fat storage: when we have an excess of glucose that is not being used for energy, our body can turn this excess glucose into fat.

The problem arises when we consume too many refined carbohydrates (pies, pastries, cakes), sugary carbonated drinks or fruit juice, or even larger portions of healthy carbs (potatoes or rice) than our body can handle. You see, the more carbohydrates we eat, the more insulin our pancreas will make. If we produce lots and lots of insulin, then the 'lock' on the cell door gets sticky (resists the action of insulin) and it is harder for the glucose to enter the cell. Our body wants to help the glucose get into the cells, so our pancreas makes even more insulin (hyperinsulinemia). As glucose is an energy source to keep our cells functioning, when it is unable to enter our cells we can start to feel fatigued and reach for something sweet for a quick pick-me-up. When insulin levels in the blood are high, this also stops 'fat-burning', meaning that fat stores are prevented from being broken down to be used for energy.

This is called insulin resistance and can set us up for a vicious cycle, as illustrated by the following diagram:

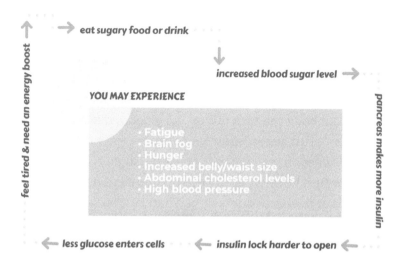

Insulin resistance syndrome, metabolic syndrome and syndrome X are some of the names used to describe a group of five warning signs (including an increased waist measurement) that we may be at risk of health problems ahead. As perimenopausal women have a one-in-three risk of developing metabolic syndrome, which increases their likelihood of developing diabetes type 2 and heart disease, the time to start taking action is now.

How can I know if I am an unhealthy weight?

So how can you tell if you may have too much visceral fat? The most accurate way to check this is to have a DEXA body composition scan. DEXA stands for dual energy X-ray absorptiometry, which will reveal your body composition of bone, muscle and visceral fat. However, not everyone can easily access or afford this type of scan, so another option is to step onto a set of body composition weight scales that will give you a breakdown of your weight into muscle mass (which burns those calories), bone mass, body fat percentage, total body water percentage and visceral fat.

The simplest and cheapest clue to whether your visceral fat may be of concern is to use a tape measure to check your waist circumference.

How can I measure my waistline?
The way to correctly measure your waist is to:

1. place a tape measure against bare skin or light-weight clothing,
2. measure at the point midway between your lowest rib and the top of your hipbone, in line with your belly button, and
3. breathe out normally.

In Australia, a Caucasian woman is at increased risk if her waist measures ≥ 80 cm (31.5 inches) and high risk if ≥ 88 cm (34.5 inches). Waist circumference for the diagnosis of abdominal obesity[13] does not uniformly apply to all populations and ethnic groups. The table below shows that a waist measurement associated high risk of metabolic syndrome[14] can vary between different ethnic groups.

Group	Waist circumference associated with high risk of metabolic syndrome
European/North American	≥ 88cm
Central & South American	≥ 80cm
Asian	≥ 80 cm
Middle Eastern/Mediterranean	≥ 80 cm
Sub-Saharan African	≥ 80 cm

Body mass index (BMI)

BMI is a ratio of weight to height for adults 18 years and over which is commonly used as a general health indicator. The normal BMI range is 18.5 to 24.9 (see following table). However, there are exceptions where this measurement is not accurate. Although a good general indicator when researchers look at population studies, athletes, who have a higher-than-average amount of lean muscle, would be incorrectly considered obese. BMI may underestimate body fat in older people. A healthy BMI tends to be lower for people of Asian ethnicity and higher for Polynesian people.

The way to calculate your BMI is to divide your weight in kilograms by your height in metres squared.

Weight (in kilograms) ÷ height (in metres, squared)

For example: If your weight is 70 kg and your height is 170 cm then your BMI = 70 ÷ (1.70 x 1.70) = 24.2

There are several easy-to-use online BMI calculators such as the one on the Australian Heart Foundation website. All you need to do is plug in your numbers and the answer will be available to compare with the chart below.

Classification	BMI
Underweight	Below 18.5
Normal	18.5 - 24.9
Overweight	25.0 - 29.9
Obesity	30.0 and above

How can I know if I have metabolic syndrome?

Firstly, grab a tape measure to check your waist measurement.

Secondly, have your blood pressure checked. It is easy enough to visit your local pharmacy and have a blood pressure check there. Another option is to take your blood pressure at home. Many people purchase or hire a machine to be able to do so.

Here are a few tips to think about when you take your own blood pressure:

* Measure your blood pressure around the same time morning and night.
* Sit quietly for five minutes without talking or watching television.
* Sit with your feet flat on the floor, legs uncrossed, and arm supported on a table or pillow so your blood pressure cuff is at heart level.
* Do not smoke or drink caffeine at least 30 minutes before taking your blood pressure.
* Take your blood pressure twice at one minute apart and record the second measurement.

Thirdly, book an appointment with your doctor to have a blood test because you will need to know your numbers to work out if you meet the criteria for metabolic syndrome.

Your blood tests will include:

* a fasting glucose test (to check your blood sugar level)
* total cholesterol
* HDL (good cholesterol)
* LDL (bad cholesterol)
* triglycerides.

If you meet three out of five of the following criteria, then this is diagnostic of metabolic syndrome:

- increased waist circumference
- elevated triglycerides ≥ 1.7 mmol/L (150 mg/dL), or you are taking medication for high triglycerides
- decreased HDL cholesterol < 1.3mmol/L (50mg/dL) in women.
- increased blood pressure ≥ 130 systolic or ≥ 85 diastolic, or you are taking medication for high blood pressure
- elevated fasting glucose ≥ 5.6 mmol/L (≥ 100 mg/dL), or you have been previously diagnosed with type 2 diabetes.

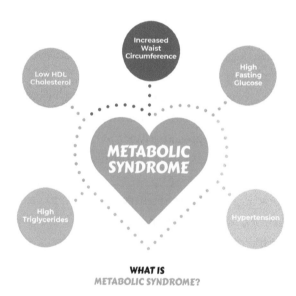

WHAT IS
METABOLIC SYNDROME?

And finally, some good news

Metabolic syndrome is reversible. You may be interested to know that the US SWAN study, which we talked about earlier, looked at whether it is possible for perimenopausal women to prevent or reverse metabolic syndrome and decrease their likelihood of developing these associated chronic health issues. The answer was YES.

If we are an unhealthy weight, or are carrying too much belly fat, then losing five to ten per cent of our total body weight can result in significant health benefits such as lowering your blood pressure, improving your blood glucose levels and reducing the risk of pushing towards diabetes, as well as helping you to feel more comfortable in your clothes.

To achieve and sustain weight loss we need to ensure we E.A.T. right. E.A.T. stands for Eating, Activity and Thinking. It is not only a matter of losing weight in the short term, but also keeping the weight off in the longer term. This requires dietary modification, physical activities to maintain lean muscle mass and improve insulin receptor sensitivity, and a change in our way of thinking to achieve sustained behaviour changes.

What can I do to reduce my middle tyre?
E is for Eating
Journalist Michael Pollan famously said that everything he has learned about food and health could be summarised in seven simple words: "Eat food, not too much, mostly plants."

"Eat food, not too much." I hate to break it to you, Jo, but in a woman's world, size does matter and the question here is: are today's food serving sizes too much of a good thing? Over the last twenty years, not only are we being dished up bigger slices of cake and portions of pizza that have added a whopping 66 per cent increase in kilojoules/kilocalories to our weight and waistlines, but our plates have been up-sized as well. Another question is: do we eat because we are hungry? Or do we eat because food is sitting on the plate in front of us?

Well might we consider the wisdom of the 2,500-year-old Confucian mantra *hara hachi bu*, which means to stop eating when our stomach is 80 per cent full. The people of Okinawa, Japan, who live by this practice, are among the longest-living people on the planet, with lower rates of chronic diseases. They generally lead healthy, vital lives with an average BMI of 18–22 (overweight is BMI > 24.9; obese is BMI > 30). Pushing away from the table when you are 80 per cent full means eating fewer calories.

You may also want to consider what you are drinking. We often don't think that fruit juice, sugary drinks, caffeinated beverages and alcohol can add a lot of calories to our daily intake, kilos to our weight and centimetres to our waist. That 250 mL glass of fruit juice at breakfast added six teaspoons of sugar to your daily intake; the 300 mL flavoured milk had seven teaspoons and the 600 mL energy drink to get you through the mid-afternoon slump added an extra eight and a half teaspoons of sugar[15]. And then there is alcohol. There have been mixed reviews about whether alcohol adds to our weight gain, with reports that heavy drinking and drinking spirits are the main problems. Generally, one gram of alcohol adds 29 kilojoules, or 7.1 kilocalories, to your intake without adding any beneficial nutrients. And often there are the nuts, chips and other nibbles we eat at the same time. OK, alcohol is a social lubricant, a relaxing shoes-off accompaniment after a challenging day, but …

At a recent information evening, I invited three people from the audience who enjoyed a red wine at night to come forward and pour from a bottle (of red coloured water) the amount of alcohol they would cuddle up with each evening.

One of the women in her mid-forties said that the wine glass provided was way too small.

"I need more of a fishbowl," she scoffed. "And I usually have at least two glasses every night."

I placed a much larger glass in front of her. "Yep, that's more like it."

Australian Alcohol Guidelines recommend 100 mL of red wine as one standard drink, but what tends to happen is that the pour-line for an average wine is more like a generous 160 mL, which is equivalent to 1.6 standard servings of red wine[16]. We calculated this lady was drinking what amounted to six standard alcoholic drinks a day and adding a whopping 485–495 calories to her daily energy intake. This lady was shocked.

Many people in the audience were shocked, too – shocked by how much they underestimated the amount of alcohol they drank, and shocked by the number of calories they were taking in.

To gain 0.5 to 1.0 kg per week you only need to be consuming an extra 500 calories per day that you are not burning off. Alcohol enhances the reward/pleasure centre in our brain and increases our appetite for food[17]. The other downside is that women who drink alcohol also increase their risk of breast cancer. According to the World Cancer Research Fund[18], there is evidence to suggest that drinking alcohol significantly increases the risk of developing breast cancer in pre-menopausal and post-menopausal women. I am not saying you shouldn't drink alcohol at all, but I suggest being considerate about how much and how often you enjoy a tipple.

"**Mostly plants.**" If you were to start by changing just one thing, I would suggest you eat your greens. Australian healthy-eating guidelines[19] recommend a woman of perimenopausal age (45–65 years) eat a minimum of five serves of different colourful vegetables and two pieces of fruit each day. A serve of vegetables is equivalent to one cup of raw, leafy greens or half a cup of cooked. Non-starchy vegetables such as broccoli, cauliflower, green beans, spinach and zucchini, and fruits such as apples, pears and berries are low (calorie) density foods due to their high-water content. They are also fibre-rich which means it takes a longer time to chew and digest them, which gives the brain time to receive the message from the gut that we feel full and satisfied. Unfortunately, only about 7 per cent of Australian women meet this daily minimum. It is important that we remember to eat enough of our greens each day – and our reds, yellows and blues ...

When someone is considering how best to reduce their weight, the question they often ask is which diet is the best one to follow. And the answer? It depends. When it comes to weight loss, there is no one-size-fits-all diet. In my experience, the most effective diet is the one that will not only help you lose weight but also keep it off.

Researchers who compared 14 different popular diets[20] found that most participants who followed the different eating patterns reported measurable weight loss at six months, along with improvement in heart health, especially in terms of reducing blood pressure. The low-carbohydrate (Atkins, Zone), low-fat (Ornish) and moderate macronutrient (Mediterranean, DASH) diets had similar weight loss results at the six-month mark. Healthy eating plans such as the Mediterranean diet and DASH (Dietary Approaches to Stop Hypertension) diet are lifelong healthy eating patterns that are prescribed by medical practitioners as nutritional therapies for the prevention and treatment of chronic health conditions. In this particular study, while weight loss was achieved at six months in all diets, after

12 months it was found the Mediterranean diet also offered long-term benefits for heart health and a lowered risk of developing Type 2 diabetes compared with all the other diets.

We are all different, so each of our metabolic machinery works slightly differently. When you embark on a nutritional, healthy eating pattern it needs to be tailored individually for your needs and the bottom line is that the best 'diet' for you is the one you will stick with. Many women follow the do-it-yourself option while others will benefit from discussing their weight loss plan with a health professional, such as an accredited dietician or nutritionist.

A is for Activity

One of the positive findings from the study is that the women who continued their regular physical exercise programs and those who increased how much exercise they were doing were able to prevent weight gain or reduce the amount of weight they gained. The physical activity included walking and riding a bike for transportation. They also reduced the amount of time they spent watching television.

Great news. So how much physical activity do we need to be doing? In Australia, exercise guidelines[21] recommend at least 30 minutes of moderate physical activity such as brisk walking (at a speed where you can talk comfortably, but not sing), swimming, dancing or cycling on at least five days a week, and at least two days a week with your exercise time allocated to resistance training to help maintain lean muscle (which helps burn calories at rest) and build core strength to keep us fit and strong.

For some reason we tend to think of physical activity as joining a team sport or training to be a triathlete but that is not necessarily the case. You may be interested to know that some of the world's longest-living, vibrant and healthy people don't go to gyms to lift weights or join a Zumba class; they simply move more as a natural part of their way of life. If you have not read Dan Buettner's book *The Blue Zones*[22] on lessons for living a healthy, active life well into your nineties, then I highly recommend you do so.

Physical activity means moving your muscles and can be as simple as doing the housework, getting down and dirty in the garden, taking the stairs instead of the lift, parking the car further away from the shopping centre entrance and returning the shopping trolley to the trolley bay, to achieve 2.5 to 5 hours of moderate huff-and-puff activity per week.

The main thing to remember is that any exercise is better than no exercise at all. If you are not in the habit of exercise, you may like to start with some simple stretching exercises to warm up, followed by walking for 10 minutes out in the fresh air or on a treadmill. You can gradually build up the time to the recommended amount. Don't underestimate the benefits of a brisk walk as weight-bearing exercise to improve your bone health.

Some women like the gym, while others prefer one-on-one time with a personal trainer. If pain or physical injuries are a limiting factor, then you might60 consider seeing an exercise physiologist who can perform an assessment and design an individual program for you.

T is for Thinking

We now understand that to reach the goal of becoming healthy, it is necessary to create a negative energy balance; that is, ENERGY IN is less than ENERGY OUT. The way to do that is by changing our dietary and physical activity habits. There are a number of self-monitoring activities that have been demonstrated to increase success in weight loss[23]: regular weighing in, using a pedometer or app to count our steps with a goal of reaching more than 10,000 steps a day, enhancing our mindful food choices by keeping a daily food log and engaging in high-intensity activity.

But what about keeping weight off in the long term? How do we resist those powerful sugar cravings? How do we deal with those destructive behaviours of eating all the foods we know we shouldn't be eating when we haven't achieved short-term weight loss? And how do we deal with our 'What's the point?' thinking when we have self-sabotaged and are teetering on the 'Will I or won't I bother' edge?

In the long run, restrictive diets alone do not work. What do I mean by that? There are many diets that help you achieve a short-term weight loss, it is the maintaining that weight loss that often proves challenging. Our ability to keep the weight off comes down to changing our mindset, and establishing and maintaining healthy lifestyle habits.

When I talk with women who want to lose those extra kilos, I suggest that they start by changing just one thing: a 'tweak a week' to establish some new positive routine rituals and not feel overwhelmed by trying to do lots of things all at once. Let me share with you a couple of examples of how effective changing just one thing can be.

KELLY

Kelly (47), a mother of three, had just completed a university degree and wanted to lose 20 kg to improve her health. This is her story:

"A year ago, I graduated. After a difficult four years I had done it, but it had taken its toll on my mental health and general wellbeing. I was miserable. At 87.9 kg I was at my heaviest weight. This morning I weighed in at 59.8 kg – the first time I have seen a five in front of my weight for 12 long years. I'm feeling better than ever and they were such simple and achievable changes and goals that I set for myself throughout this past year. In fact, it didn't cost me a cent apart from my new Fitbit watch and a pair of supportive joggers. There was no gym, no fad diets, no pills or potions, no outside help. I knew I could do it, so I did. And how did I start? I began by making one small change: to cut out junk food. My next step, literally, was to start walking and working up to 10,000 steps at least five days a week. Then I started to jog and I have not looked back."

JULIET

Juliet (46), a project manager, found a simple way to stop undermining her mindful eating habits:

"I found that I was in the habit of eating something sweet after dinner. Every day I was mindful about what I was eating but at night I was self-sabotaging my efforts. Chocolate was my weakness. Every night I would promise myself that I'd only eat a couple of squares of dark choco-late because I had heard that dark chocolate was OK, but I would end up eating the whole bar. And then I'd feel really cross with myself because in a few minutes I'd just undone all the good stuff I'd done during the day. Then I decided to clean my teeth immediately after eating my

evening meal and that was the game changer for me. I associated cleaning my teeth with not eating afterwards and now I have achieved my weight loss goal and two years down the track I am maintaining my weight. Who would have thought that something so simple would be that effective? But it works for me."

Establishing healthy habits

Sometimes it is not simply the fact of losing weight but keeping it off. Personalised cognitive behavioural therapy[24] (CBT) looks at how our thoughts (cognition) can influence our feelings and unhealthy behaviours. It can also be used to help with problems in our relationship with food. A practitioner works with each individual to develop practical strategies to overcome the obstacles to weight loss in the short term, as well as maintaining a sustainable weight in the longer term. As you can see from the diagram below, thoughts, feelings and behaviours are all interlinked.

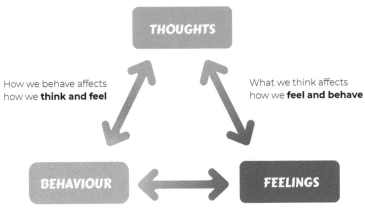

It is important when we do slip up and succumb to a binge or don't make that weight loss goal to exercise self-compassion and realise that we all slip up from time to time. A relapse does not inactivate all of our achievements. Smokers commonly make several attempts to quit before they can kick their habit and we recognise it is a relapse, not a failure.

If you would like some help in this area, your doctor can write you a referral to a certified dietician, psychologist or counsellor skilled in this area, who is able to empower you to identify what triggers your weight-gain mindset and work out practical strategies to prevent setbacks.

If you are struggling with weight management, please reach out for the assistance and support you need to make those changes. Making meaningful changes today in things you do have power over, in my opinion, is a form of real health insurance to become the best version of yourself now for your future self, twenty, thirty or forty years from now.

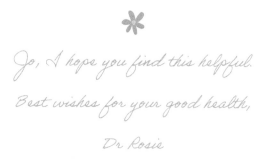

Jo, I hope you find this helpful.

Best wishes for your good health,

Dr Rosie

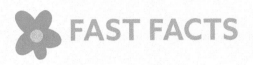 **FAST FACTS**

Why do many midlife women gain weight?

It is an often mistaken believe that weight gain is simply due to a
lack of willpower however, this is not the case. There are several
different reasons for midlife weight gain that have little to do
with willpower such as increasing age, genetics, the epigenetic
effect of environmental factors that switch on or switch off genes,
hormones, sleep deprivation, gut microbiota, inflammation, lack
of physical activity and certain medications.

Why is gaining weight around my middle a problem?

Apart from not being able to zip up your favourite skinny jeans,
it seems that as our waist measurement increases, so too, do
our health risks. A larger waist measurement is associated with
abdominal obesity and visceral fat. Some researchers have
called this excess visceral fat 'sick fat' as it plays havoc with our
metabolic rate and makes us put on weight more easily, especially
around the middle. A larger waist measurement is one of five
warning signs of possible metabolic syndrome.

How can I know if I have metabolic syndrome?

Metabolic syndrome describes a cluster of five symptoms which
includes an increased waist measurement. As perimenopausal
women have a one-in-three risk of developing metabolic
syndrome, which increases their likelihood of developing diabetes
type 2 and heart disease, the time to start taking action is now.
The good news is that metabolic syndrome is preventable and

reversible. Weight gain and serious health problems are not inevitable.

How can I reduce my middle tyre?

If we are an unhealthy weight, or are carrying too much belly fat, then a modest weight loss of 5 to 10 per cent of our total body weight can result in significant health benefits as well as helping us feel comfortable in our clothes. To achieve weight loss and maintain a healthy weight requires a combination of physical activities to maintain lean muscle mass and improve insulin receptor sensitivity, dietary and behaviour changes.

Chapter 4
MOOD SWINGS

Men-o-pause!

In 1821 a French physician, Charles-somebody-or-other, came up with the word *menopause*. While the official story is that it's the combination of two Greek works – *pausis*, meaning pause and *mēn*, meaning month – I can't help but wonder if Charles had a wife who was pissing him off!

It's an interesting word when you consider it – MEN-O-PAUSE! Is it a time for us to pause from men? This may have been the case in Charles' world and I'm sure there are men all around the world who would love to pause from their wives and partners whilst they navigate their way through 'the change'.

In an ideal world, wouldn't it be awesome if we could take a pause from everyone and everything? Imagine if there was a designated place where we were sent (and no, not a mental asylum), a retreat to convalesce, considering some of us may have recently completed or are currently undertaking the 30 years of hard, painstaking labour of raising a family. LIFE-PAUSE would be more fitting at this time. I find 'change of life' has unsavoury connotations of irrelevance and being past one's use-by date – an insulting phrase that could attract a punch in the face to anyone who dares to use it. A male client recently suggested that I must be going through the 'change of life' because I was the same age as his mother. And then proceeded to tell me that his dad had told him that all women go crazy at this time; it was like waving a red flag in front of a bull. Lucky for him, he wasn't charged and taken out! In this case, 'death by change' would be more appropriate.

I've noticed I'm less tolerant these days; I feel irritated A LOT! Many things irritate me that never irritated me before. Once upon a time I would have put myself out for anybody, anything, anytime; not now, I just can't be bothered. Attending functions, events and special occasions that I would have once fussed about are now an effort and can often cause stress and discomfort. It's not that I don't care, but I feel like I don't have the time to waste on what can sometimes be trivial, tiresome commitments.

I'm sure a lot of my irritation is caused by lack of quality sleep. I've always loved to sleep. Sleeping has been my saviour: a place of warmth and peace. My once-perfect sleeping pattern is now interrupted, which makes for a very irritable following day. The smallest problem appears 10 times greater at 2 am and I create mountains out of molehills. My stress levels are heightened, and I'm overwhelmed with anxiety and feel alone. It's no surprise I am now being medicated for high blood pressure.

You could also say I'm a little *snappy*. I recently brought snapdragon flowers into the house and my husband said, "We don't need any more snapdragons; we already have one is this house!" We looked at each other and roared with laughter – he was lucky he got me on a good day.

My personality is changing, and I am learning the art of not giving a f**k. I often feel unemotional while at other times highly emotional, just like having PMT constantly, not just once a month. I'm on this crazy rollercoaster: up, down, round and round, hot, cold, exhausted, frustrated, tired and irritated. I don't indulge in alcohol, but I understand how one could find solace in getting drunk and passing out.

It's easy to throw another biscuit in your mouth when your self-esteem is low, and you feel ripped off, pissed off and out of control. I now know why I hate the phrase 'change of life' because I wasn't prepared for what would change. And now I'm here, I'm irritable (yep, in case you hadn't noticed) and incredibly sad.

I'm deeply depressed and feel like I'm grieving a loss – the loss of a former level-headed, adaptable, always happy, sociable well-slept me! My greatest sanity is yoga. Thank God for yoga or I may have killed someone by now. Apparently, if you don't have time for an hour of yoga, you should do two!

As much as it's exciting to become empty-nesters and to turn the next page, it also highlights the end of a chapter: the conclusion of raising children and caring for a family. It's easy to feel obsolete when you're not essential.

We can't blame our mothers for this lack of ignorance and understanding of menopause – or can we? Some have died before their daughters hit menopause and others are of the generation where you just sucked it up and got on with it. When I consider it, my mother had her own struggles with depression, which was heightened during this time. She never warned me of what to expect and, of course, I never under-stood what she was going through at the time as I was too wrapped up in my own world to notice. Imagine if my Dad had said, "It's OK, Mum's just finding herself as a new woman, so she's taking a pause from me, you, your brothers and sister and life in general at the moment. We just need to give her some space (maybe ten years!)"

My Dad would never have had this discussion with me. He was no sensitive, new-age guy; he was old-school and never spoke about anything to do with our bodies – that was Mum's domain. I'm sure he had no clear understanding of what Mum was going through; her change of moods, antisociality and attitude would have been put down to depression – and she may have been hospitalised. Now that I look back, my Dad played a lot of golf then and he was always at the golf club when I called home. He played most days, often twice a day, and definitely drank a lot more beer.

I would have been grateful had someone – anyone – explained it in this context: "I know this is hard to believe, but one day you might become this crazy, psycho bitch whose head would spin around a few times a day, and you might release a little verbal diarrhoea on the world that will more than likely offend someone. You won't be apologetic or expect retaliation for your actions because it's OK – that's just what happens!"

Dear Dr Rosie,

I've noticed I'm much less tolerant than I
once was. I feel irritated. A LOT! And I get
moody, and cranky and easily frustrated and
sometimes I feel down in the dumps and —did I
mention it? — IRRITATED!

- Is it normal to feel irritable and moody, as
  if I have PMS 24/7?
- Are there specific perimenopause or
  menopause counsellors?
- Is there anything I can do to reduce the
  stress I feel?

Thanks,
Jo

Let's talk about mood swings

Hi Jo,

I heard the rawness and power of your upset and frustration in your last letter. Thank you for your honesty because what your experience is a variation on the theme of what many women experience: the exasperation that at times their body is behaving like some sort of physical and emotional out-of-control rollercoaster, the upset that no one gave them a heads-up on what might be happening, and the frustration of not knowing whether there is anything they can do to make a difference to the way they are feeling. Let's have a chat about all of that.

Is it normal to feel irritable and moody, as if I have PMS 24/7?

As it happens, feelings of anxiety, irritability, crankiness, annoyance, impatience, and those momentary outbursts of anger, are common during the perimenopausal transition phase. In fact, a review of several different international studies found that irritability can occur in up to 70 per cent[1] of perimenopausal women in many different regions of the globe. Thankfully, scientific research confirms that those emotional ups and downs will settle with time.

Fluctuating hormone levels and mood swings

Although oestrogen is best known as a sex hormone, it also nourishes and protects our brain structure and functioning[2]. Oestrogen and progesterone influence the serotonin 'happy hormone' pathways in our brain, which affect mood. Oestrogen also has an effect on both our memory and emotional centres in the brain – the hippocampus and amygdala – which helps us to judge and respond to social and environmental situations going on around us.

Scientists suggest that it is the dramatic, erratic hormone fluctuations which contribute to mood swings and depressive symptoms, making us feel like we are riding some emotional roller coaster, rather than simply the eventual declining oestrogen level as a woman transitions into menopause[3]. Further, research[4] suggested that dramatic hormonal swings may be a contributing factor to lower moods in a sample of perimenopausal women who did not have depressive symptoms.

Remember, we previously talked about how during the perimenopause, our ovaries can release oestrogen erratically, with oestradiol (E2) levels sometimes going up high and at other times dropping very low[5]. Scientists have found that perimenopausal women experience significantly higher hormonal 'highs' and much lower 'lows' of oestrogen compared with women of younger reproductive age. Thankfully, hormones levels become more stable and settled after menopause.

In fact, there has been increasing recognition that perimenopause is a time 'window of vulnerability' for the development of a new or recurrent episode of depression. Depression is more common during perimenopause, in fact the risk of developing a new mood disorder is 30 to 60 per cent higher[6] during this transition time compared with pre- or post-menopausal years. Those who are most at risk during this timeframe include those who have previously experienced depression, premenstrual syndrome (PMS) and postnatal depression (PND). Now, let me make the distinction here that being at risk does not necessarily mean you will experience another depressive episode. It is a bit like travelling in a car. You are at greater risk of having a motor vehicle accident if you go out driving in a car compared to staying at home. Being at risk when you go out in the car does not necessarily mean you will have an accident. In the same way, the fact that you have had a previous episode of a depressive illness does not necessarily mean you will have another episode at this stage of your life. However, it is a matter of being aware.

Mood swings, irritability, sleep disturbances, weight gain and fatigue are all menopausal symptoms which can overlap with depression.

There is no blood test or imaging scan to diagnose a depressive disorder, which is why it is called a disorder or illness and not a disease, but this is definitely something not to be ignored. Symptoms of depression can impact our functioning and include:

* persistent feelings of sadness, feelings of emptiness
* irritability, anger or frustration over seemingly little things

- little interest or loss of interest in activities or hobbies that were once pleasurable
- disturbed sleep, insomnia, early-morning waking or sleeping a lot
- change in appetite with either a decreased or increased appetite
- fatigue, a lack of energy
- difficulty concentrating
- feelings of worthlessness or excessive guilt
- frequent or recurring thoughts about death or suicide.

So, if you are not feeling your usual self, behaving out of character, or experiencing any of the symptoms of depression, there are a couple of questions to ask yourself:

- Over the past two weeks, have you felt down, depressed or hopeless?
- Over the past two weeks, have you felt little interest or pleasure in doing things?

If you find that you answered yes to either question, and/or have experienced any of the symptoms listed above more than occasionally, then I suggest you make an appointment with your doctor. It is important to be assessed individually as there is no one-size-fits-all solution. Some of the treatment options considered may include counselling, mindfulness-based[7] exercise programs and relaxation techniques; medication may or may not be indicated. Sometimes it can be tricky to untangle things because there are several issues other than hormones going on that also need to be addressed.

Hormones are only one piece of the puzzle

It would be easy to point the finger and suggest that the fluc-tuating, and ultimately declining, levels of oestrogen are solely responsible for increased irritability and mood swings. Whilst changing hormone levels certainly play a part, the reality is that hormonal changes are only one piece of the puzzle that may be influencing our moods. Let me explain. Women in midlife are often positioned as 'the meat in the sandwich' having to deal with issues involving two different generations: youth on one side and aging parents on the other side. Additionally, it is possible that midlife women may be dealing with their own physical health problems, work-related issues or relationship concerns. As you may now appreciate, physical, psychological factors may contribute to our mood.

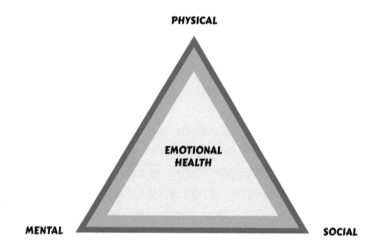

The World Health Organisation defines health as "a state of complete physical, mental and social well-being and not merely the absence of disease"[8]. This includes mental health because our physical, psychological and social wellbeing will affect how we think, how we feel and how we behave. We find that if any one area or any combination of these different areas becomes disrupted, then the disruption(s) can affect our overall functioning and quality of life. Hormones are one of the physical factors. Let's have a look at some other physical factors that may be contributing to our emotional health.

Physical factors

Distress associated with physical menopause symptoms

A perimenopausal woman may be struggling with physical discomfort associated with hot flushes, night sweats, disrupted sleep and low libido, as well as a difficulty to concentrate and mood swings. Whether caused by a snoring partner, worries circling around and around in her head like a broken record as soon as her head hits the pillow, disruptive hot flushes and 'throw the covers off' night sweats alternating with 'now I need the covers back on' chills, or trying to get some shut-eye in a noisy environment, a room that is not dark enough, waking unrefreshed and tired can really impact her mood and erode her tolerance.

Medical conditions

Have you ever crawled into bed with a nasty dose of the flu? Your body feels achy, you want to sleep, don't feel like eating, your mood feels flat and you certainly don't want to socialise. This usually short-term sickness behaviour is because your body's immune system has ramped up its production of inflammatory molecules to fight off the invading infection[9]. What might happen if this turned out to become a long-term inflammatory condition? Any medical condition that ends with -itis has an inflammatory component. Research has demonstrated that inflammation anywhere in the body is associated with a depressed mood[10,11,12].

Other medical conditions that can affect our mood include a low-functioning thyroid (depressive mood) or a high-functioning thyroid (anxiety, heart palpitations, sweats) and autoimmune disorders including coeliac disease.

Prescription and recreational drugs

Another physical reason for low mood at this time may be side-effects of prescription or recreational drugs and yes, I am including alcohol here because whilst it is a relaxing social lubricant, it can also have a depressive effect. There are several medications that can affect mood. Certain prescription drugs must not be stopped suddenly, so if you think one of your medications may be messing with your mood, make sure you consult with your doctor to see if there are other treatment options.

Nutritional deficiencies

Low levels of certain vitamins such as B_{12}, iron, folate and vitamin D are also associated with low mood or depression[13], so it is important to eliminate whether you have such deficiencies by having a blood test.

Psychological factors

Although menopause is not an illness or a pathological disease, for some women, perimenopause can be associated with increased psychological stress. As our body changes, so too many of our beliefs regarding fertility, ageing and shifts in our social role may be reviewed and possibly challenged. Many women, as they enter into menopause, report a sense of freedom: freedom from painful, heavy or unpredictable menstrual periods; freedom from the constraints of contraception; and a renewed sense of wellbeing as they take up pursuits they had previously put on hold as they focused on fulfilling responsibilities to others. Other women may experience a sense of grief, loss or distress that their reproductive door is closing; others, as they deal with the quiet of an empty nest, changes in their body shape or serious health issues.

Whether we are feeling happy about our future or emotionally weighed down, these feelings and emotions are always associated with a set of thoughts. Sometimes we may have fallen into a pattern of thinking in unhelpful ways. Unhelpful automatic ways of thinking are usually outside of our conscious awareness but can certainly add to our emotional distress. It's like having a parrot with a bad attitude sitting on your shoulder and squawking negative things in your ear like, "You stumbled over your words in front of everyone in the meeting, you're such an idiot," (catastrophising) or "If you can't do it right the first time, then you're a failure," (black-and-white-thinking). Add to that the dramatic, erratic hormonal fluctuations and we can end up being overly self-critical and giving our self-esteem a beating. There's more information on unhelpful thinking on my website, if you'd like to learn more.

Please remember to be kind to yourself. In my experience many, many women are extremely hard on themselves, pushing themselves to be perfect. Hillary Langford first penned the 'Ten Commandments for Reducing Stress' in 1987 and I am grateful to her for allowing me to share them with you. Hilary is a fount of compassion and wisdom and can be contacted by email at mentor@hilary.com.au.

TEN COMMANDMENTS FOR REDUCING STRESS

Thou shalt:

1. not be perfect, nor even try to be.

2. not try to be all things to all people.

3. leave things undone that ought to be done.

4. not spread thyself too thin.

5. learn to say 'no'.

6. schedule time for thyself, and thy supportive network.

7. switch off and do nothing regularly.

8. be boring, untidy, inelegant and unattractive at times.

9. not even feel guilty.

10. especially not be thine own worst enemy, but be thy best friend.

Source: Used with kind permission of Hilary Langford, email at mentor@hilary.com.au

Social factors

And if that isn't enough, multiple social pressures also tend to come into play at this midlife stage. Often, women in peri-menopause are sandwiched between two generations. On one side they might have children still living at home, or are adjusting to the new role of an empty-nester; on the other side they might have ageing parents dealing with health concerns, or be dealing with the grief and loss following the death of a parent, or having to make decisions about nursing home admission(s). Commonly, women are also juggling work obligations and may have financial concerns. There may be relationship issues with their intimate partner, and they may even consider uncoupling with the realisation that their life goals are no longer aligned, leading to break-ups or divorce, and the list goes on.

Is there a hole in your bucket (dear Liza)? In my experience, many women are dipping from their energy resources, AKA their energy bucket, giving of their time and energy to others. Often, the giving is done with generosity and pleasure, but sometimes women realise that they are feeling depleted and their bucket of once-boundless energy is getting low. Is it any wonder that some women feel that their get-up-and-go has well and truly got-up-and-gone, and that they experience a lack of motivation or enthusiasm to do the things they used to find enjoyable?

Sometimes decreasing energy reserves are also further depleted by poor sleep, skipping meals and working long hours without a break. My question is: what are you doing to replenish your resources? How can we reduce the stress of overwhelm and reduced energy?

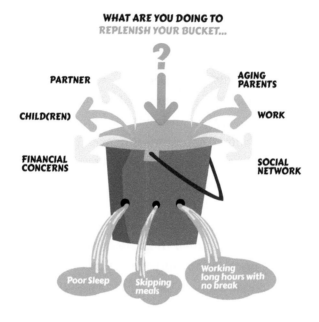

Are there specific perimenopause or menopause counsellors?

Jo, you wondered if there are specific menopause counsellors to assist women as they adjust to their new roles and challenges. Many GPs have training in psychological skills training and there are many clinical psychologists who can assist with a range of concerns that women in their middle years may have, whether it is managing physical symptoms of hot flushes and sleep disturbance, or dealing with grief, loss and low self-esteem, or with a depressive mood. For example, there is now good evidence that cognitive behavioural therapy (CBT) is an effective non-hormone-based treatment for managing physical symptoms of hot flushes, night sweats and sleep disturbance in addition to mood issues of anxiety and depression.

In Australia, your GP will talk with you to make an assessment. Following your assessment, some doctors with further training in focused psychological strategies will work with you, whereas others will refer you to a clinical psychologist or qualified counsellor for a number of face-to-face consultations or online sessions. The reason that I refer people for these sessions is not simply for debriefing and talk therapy, which, by the way, may be very beneficial, but mainly as a means to access some very practical 'tools in the toolbox' to assist you as you navigate your journey.

Is there anything I can do to reduce the stress I feel?

Although stress is a natural response in dealing with demanding situations, it becomes tricky when we feel overwhelmed. We all tend to look at situations through the filters of our personality and previous experiences: what one person considers to be stressful, another might view as an insurmountable challenge. Some of the strategies to reduce stress that I have found to be helpful include:

Don't overschedule. I used to be guilty of trying to pack more into my day than I could comfortably deal with until I realised that I could not squeeze everything on my 'to do' list into my day. Having admitted that it is not possible to do everything, the next step is to:

Prioritise your tasks. Determine what is urgent and important, and what is important but not so urgent. Once you have decided what needs doing and when, commit to giving your full attention to the task at hand.

Schedule personal time out. All work and no play ... It may be as simple as taking 20 minutes to curl up with a cup of tea, spending time in some green space, going for a walk in the fresh air or catching up with friends.

If you use a hardcopy diary, I recommend scheduling time out each day for yourself and writing it in pen, which means it is non-negotiable. Commitments to all other people and events are written in pencil as this can be changed. Now in the day of electronic calendaring, CAPITALISE YOUR TIME OUT and lowercase everyone else's time.

Relax your mind, relax your body. Mindful meditation has been shown to help reduce our reactivity to stress and improving our resilience[14,15]. Yoga[16,17], tai chi[18], and qigong are traditional mind-body therapies that assist with improving our emotional and physical wellbeing.

Remember to breathe. Breathing is essential to life. And when we are exercising, or laughing, or feeling anxious and stressed, our breathing can change and have a physical effect on the way we feel. For example, have you ever started an exercise program that involved climbing stairs and felt fatigued and out of breath, only to find yourself, when doing the same exercise a few weeks later, racing up those stairs two at a time and feeling strong and not the least bit out of breath?

When we feel stressed, we tend to take faster, shallower breaths and our chest muscles become tensed and tight. This is the 'fight, flight or freeze' response when stress hormones and the sympathetic nervous system go into overdrive. Although breathing is automatic, we can have some control over the way we breathe, which will decrease our body's stress response. Slower, deeper 'belly breathing' (commonly called diaphragmatic breathing) can relax our body and calm our mind. I remember an only son with social anxiety who had to speak at his father's funeral in front of an expected 200 people. His voice shook, his hands shook, his body trembled, and he had that 'deer-in-the-headlights' terror as he described his upcoming ordeal and asked for Valium. I said, "Instead of the Valium, how about you learn a skill that will be just as effective and help your through other times in the future when you feel anxious or panicky?"

We sat together and practised what I call 'Blue Belly Breathing', also known as Four-by-Four Breathing, together. This is the technique:

Start by visualising a blue square (see diagram on the next page). Hold your hands under the bottom of your ribs, relax your belly and starting at the TOP LEFT side of the square, breathe in for the count of four; from TOP RIGHT to BOTTOM RIGHT, hold your breath for the count of four; working your way across from BOTTOM RIGHT to BOTTOM LEFT, breathe out for the count of four; and working your way up from BOTTOM LEFT to TOP LEFT, hold for the count of four. Repeat the cycle for a couple of minutes. It works. There are lots of different variations on this theme. Deep belly breathing engages the diaphragm and activates the parasympathetic part of our nervous system to slow our heart rate and lower blood pressure[19].

A couple of weeks later, the young man called me to say that the breathing technique had really helped him. He had made it through the eulogy with not a tremor in his voice or hands, and many people congratulated him on his poise.

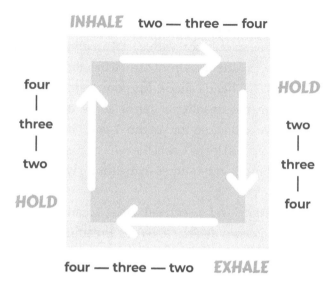

INHALE   two — three — four

four
|
three
|
two

HOLD

HOLD

two
|
three
|
four

four — three — two   EXHALE

SARAH

Sarah (49), an office manager, admitted that stress was contributing to her hot flushes and often her life felt out of control as she tried to keep up with her non-stop, crazy, busy schedule.

"I was in this spiral of playing catch-up with my life. I had this massive list of things to do, and I was caught up in the urgency of ticking boxes for everyone else so there didn't seem to be any time left for me to look after me. I wasn't even on my own list of things to do. I knew I needed to do something but doing something for me just felt like one more thing to do on my already long 'to do' list."

Sarah committed to five minutes of deep belly breathing at the beginning of each day.

"I remembered that a few years ago I used to have half an hour of yoga and meditation practice and how good I felt. Taking time out for a simple five minutes' meditative breathing practice seemed almost beyond my capacity; however, I had made a commitment to myself that I was going to make scheduling time for myself a priority. As soon as I started, I wondered why I had avoided doing this sooner. After a few days I found that doing five minutes of breathing really made a difference to helping me get my head together. That one simple change was a game changer."

Physical activity and being mindful about what we eat, reducing our caffeine intake, not overdoing alcohol as it has a depressive effect in large amounts, getting sufficient restorative sleep, and maintaining a connection with a supportive network of family and friends are all important to consider for mental wellbeing.

Jo, I know there has been a lot to take in as we have discussed how our mood can be influenced by physical, social and psychological factors. Perhaps this information will give you a better understanding of what you are experiencing and why you are feeling the way you do. I hope these tips for making some positive changes will help you gain a greater sense of control in your life. Finally, a gentle reminder to have a chat with your doctor if you need a referral to a psychologist to learn some practical 'tools in your toolbox'.

Jo, I hope you find this helpful.

Best wishes for your good health,

Dr Rosie

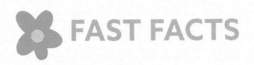 **FAST FACTS**

Is it normal to feel irritable and moody, as if I have PMS 24/7?

As it happens, feelings of anxiety, irritability, crankiness, annoyance, impatience and those momentary outbursts of anger are common during the perimenopausal transition phase. In fact, a review of several international studies found that irritability can occur in up to 70 per cent of perimenopausal women in many different regions of the globe.

Are there specific perimenopause or menopause counsellors?

There are many GPs who have extra training and expertise in providing focused psychological strategies as well as qualified clinical psychologists and certified counsellors who can assist with a range of concerns that women in their middle years encounter.

Is there anything I can do to reduce the stress I feel?

- Don't overschedule.
- Prioritise your tasks.
- Schedule personal time.
- Relax your mind, relax your body. Mindful meditation has been demonstrated to have a positive effect on certain parts of our brain by reducing our reactivity to stress and improving our resilience. Yoga, tai chi, and qigong are traditional mind–body therapies that assist with improving our emotional and physical wellbeing.

❋ Remember to breathe. Deep belly breathing engages our diaphragm and activates the parasympathetic part of the nervous system to slow the heart rate and lower blood pressure. This physical relaxation promotes physical health and mental wellbeing[20].

Chapter 5

DRY AND ITCHY SKIN

Itchy scratchy

Having suffered from eczema most of my adult life, I've spent years itching and scratching. Most of my family have spent their life telling me to STOP SCRATCHING. Which is fine for anyone who doesn't have an itch that needs scratching. Although I've learnt to manage the itch, the flaking skin has plagued my existence and caused a nuisance in my car, bed, clothes and lounge. Anywhere I have stopped long enough, remnants of myself have been left in evidence, making the job of any future CSI so much easier – how gross!

Some of my girlfriends are experiencing dry, itchy skin for the first time. They explain that they feel as though ants are crawling under their skin, and they are going crazy scratching their arms, legs and scalps like mad monkeys. Some are so affected by the irritation that they scratch until they bleed and have resorted to living on antihistamines.

With eczema, I understand the cycle of dry skin. You have an irritation, so you scratch it, then because you scratch it you need to scratch it more and more until you've scratched it so much that your skin cracks and bleeds. You go through the process of repairing the broken skin by means of moisturisers and steroid creams with the hope that it doesn't get infected – until you realise you have scratched yourself silly and have affected areas all over your body, and so the cycle continues.

Recently a work colleague informed me that in the lead up menopause, not only does your vagina become desert-like but your whole body dries out. Her hair has become coarse and splits easily, making it hard to manage and style. She's also concerned about her dry mouth and ongoing dental problems. Her skin needs constant care, so moisturising her entire body has become a daily ritual. Unfortunately, her efforts are barely scratching the surface with no amount of hydration able to reverse the effects of ageing from dry skin.

My beautician friend has noticed that many of her clients in their fifties are experiencing similar dryness, especially around their eyes and lips, and therefore are turning to fillers for a quick fix. She explains that their skin loses it elasticity and becomes as thin as tissue paper, which is common on the face, neck, hands, arms, and underarms but is least noticeable on the legs. Hence why she has clients in their eighties who are still rocking great legs. She explains that our collagen and elastic fibres reduce as we age although she believes dryness and itchiness can stem from 20 years of doing little or nothing and then playing the catch-up game. She believes hydration can most definitely reverse the effects of dryness although at the end of the day stress is a major factor in the way our skin looks and feels.

There's no surprise that finding the time over the past 30 years to nurture ourselves and care for our skin may have been neglected with our priority to look after our children, partners and parents before ourselves.

So, whilst I continue to scratch myself to death, I'm

compassionate to those who are now scratching themselves senseless with an itch that just needs to be scratched!

Wow, the effects of decreasing oestrogen really do have a lot to answer for!

Dear Dr Rosie,

- Is dryness associated with 'the change' or is it just ageing?
- Why can it sometimes feel like there are ants crawling under my skin?
- Is there anything else I can do to look after my skin?

Thanks,
Jo

Let's talk about dry, itchy skin

You are touching (excuse the pun) on what seems to be an age-old concern for many women. Cleopatra was renowned for bathing in asses' milk and women in ancient Greece used olive oil and honey to keep their skin supple and smooth.

Is dry skin simply due to ageing or could declining oestrogen levels also play a role? Before answering this question, let's first have a closer look at our skin. Then we will consider the changes over time and finally, what we can do to help ourselves in the dry skin department.

Let's get acquainted with our skin

Let me introduce you to the largest organ in your body: our amazing, dynamic, living and breathing skin. If we have a closer look at our skin, we find that it is made up of three main layers. I tend to think of our skin layers as a 'skin sandwich' with the *epidermis* as the top slice of bread, the *dermis* being like the filling in the middle, and *subcutaneous tissue* representing the bottom slice. I have simplified this even more in the diagram below.

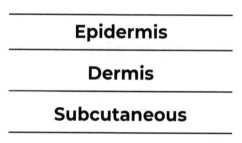

Figure: The 'Skin Sandwich' layers of the skin

The epidermis

When we look at our skin, it is the uppermost part of the epidermis, called the stratum corneum, that we see. Plump new skin cells form lower down in the basement level of this layer. As more and more new skin cells are formed, like a slow shuffle they take about one month to push upward before they reach the uppermost part of the skin. As these cells move upward, they squeeze out lipids (fatty substances). These lipids (ceramides, cholesterol and free fatty acids) act like mortar to bond the now flattened cell 'bricks' in an organised pattern. The physical bricks and the chemical mortar work together to form a protective waterproof barrier on our skin. This protective barrier prevents excessive water loss and dehydration and protects lower layers from harmful irritants, allergens, organisms, and other substances from the outside environment. Eventually, there is a natural process in which these cell 'bricks' dry out and flake off the surface of our skin, making way for new ones to replace them.

Sebum is a natural oil secreted by sebaceous glands located near the base of hair follicles which helps lubricate our skin. Many of us may have experienced oily skin and acne in our younger years but the amount of sebum that we produce also decreases over time. Our skin also makes compounds collectively called the *natural moisturising factor* (NMF), which helps keep our skin looking healthy and hydrated by attracting and holding onto water molecules. These moistening agents (or *humectants*) work by absorbing moisture from the air in humid conditions and drawing water from deeper down in the skin. NMF also maintains the normally slightly acidic pH of our skin as a barrier to microorganisms. The level of NMF decreases as we age. When we don't have enough NMF, our skin can become dry and flaky, and can even crack and split. Washing with soap strips NMF and sebum from our skin, which is why people with eczema (also known as *atopic dermatitis*), psoriasis and other dryskin conditions are advised to use a soap-free wash.

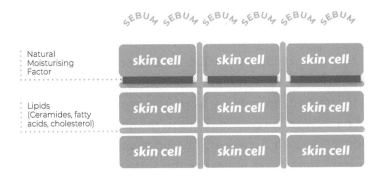

In the basement level of our epidermis we also find melanin-making cells called *melanocytes*. Melanin is a natural pigment that acts like an umbrella to protect our skin from the damaging effects of UV radiation. UVC rays are mainly absorbed by the atmospheric ozone layer, but UVB rays penetrate the epidermis where they cause sunburn, DNA damage that sets us up for skin cancers. UVA radiation penetrates even deeper into the underlying dermis, where it further damages our DNA, which can lead to more skin cancers, and contributes to premature ageing. Now, let's have a look at that 'sandwich filling' underneath the epidermis, the dermis.

The dermis

The dermis is around 20 to 30 times thicker than the epidermis above it. This layer is rich in collagen, which provides structure and support to the skin, together with thick elastic fibres which are made up of the protein elastin, that allow our skin to glide, stretch and spring back into shape[1]. Scattered throughout this layer we find nerves and a network of small blood vessels that carry nutrients to nourish the skin collagen together with water-loving *glycosaminoglycans* (GAGs), such as hyaluronic acid, that help retain moisture.

The subcutaneous layer

The lowest skin layer is mainly made up of fat cells. It plumps up our skin, insulates, cushions, and protects underlying bones and muscle. Although this layer is hidden from view, it can affect our appearance as we age, especially on our face and neck. With the passage of time, the amount of fat in this layer of our skin decreases; fine lines and hollows around our eyes and cheeks appear as the surface skin follows the changing contours of the underlying dermis and subcutaneous layers.

Is dryness associated with 'the change' or is it just ageing?

With the passage of time, our skin becomes drier as it has more difficulty holding onto moisture; decreased levels of collagen also leave skin thinner, less elastic and more prone to developing fine lines and wrinkles. So, is the dryness due to ageing, changes in hormones or the result of various environmental assaults? The ageing process in skin is a bit of a double whammy because it is caused by both intrinsic and extrinsic factors.

Intrinsic ageing

Intrinsic ageing happens from within us under the influence of our genetic inheritance and declining oestrogen levels. When considering the influence of genetics, you might ask yourself, what was your mother's skin like? To gain a more complete scientific understanding of this, researchers are continuing to look at how our genes influence skin ageing and how particular patterns of genes are 'switched on' in women who have younger-looking skin for their age[2]. So, stay tuned.

The role of oestrogen in helping to maintain smooth, hydrated skin has been more extensively studied[3] [4]. You may recall that oestrogen receptors, which are located where oestrogen works and has an effect, are spread throughout the body. It may not surprise you that a lower level of oestrogen is going to affect your skin, too. Oestrogen is involved in the production of collagen, so, as oestrogen levels decline, our skin can become thinner and less elastic, which leads to fine wrinkles. Oestrogen also plays a role in the production of natural oils, NMF and GAGs (mentioned above). Therefore, as oestrogen declines along with natural oils, the moisture in our skin also decreases and our skin becomes thinner, drier, itchy, flaky and sensitive.

That dry, itchy, sensitive skin can show up on our face, chest, back, arms and elbows, lower limbs, and genitals – and we are going to talk about dryness downstairs in a later chapter.

Extrinsic ageing

When we consider extrinsic ageing, these are the external factors and environmental influences that may contribute to our skin ageing faster than might be expected. Whilst we may have no control over certain intrinsic factors such as our genetics and changing hormone levels, we certainly can make choices about lifestyle factors that can influence extrinsic ageing. And the good news, it is never too late to start making some positive changes. I will talk about some suggestions later in this chapter.

Why can it sometimes feel like there are ants crawling under my skin?

Some women say they feel distressed by the sensation of ants crawling under their skin. In medical-speak this is called *formication*, from the Latin word for ant, *formica*. Some women say that it feels more like a tingling, pricking sensation, a bit like 'pins and needles'. Other women find it triggers an itchy feeling and all they want to do is scratch and scratch and scratch. Unfortunately, scratching can lead to an itch-and-scratch cycle, which is even worse with thinning skin because it can cause skin damage that takes longer to heal.

Lowered oestrogen levels can be associated with this sensation. Sometimes it can also happen if we suddenly stop certain medications[5]. Please have a chat with your doctor if this feeling is of concern.

Is there anything else I can do to look after my skin?

Sun exposure

From the time we are children, our facial skin is exposed to sunlight and the potentially harmful effects of UVA and UVB rays. Whilst sun exposure is important for the production of vitamin D and our emotional wellbeing, too much sun exposure can have an ageing effect and increase our risk of skin cancers, pigmented age spots and wrinkles. It has been suggested that sun exposure may be responsible for up to 80 per cent of the signs of ageing in women with Caucasian skin from the US, UK, Canada and Australia[6]. In one study[7] Australian women reported moderate to severe signs of facial ageing up to 20 years earlier than women in the US. However, this does not mean that all Australian women are ageing prematurely. Perhaps one of the main messages of this particular study is the importance of avoiding UV exposure by wearing sunscreen, a hat and other protective clothing. Get into the habit of wearing clothing that covers as much of your skin as possible, wear a hat that covers your face, head, ears and neck and, 30 minutes before you head into the sunshine, apply a broad-spectrum, water-resistant sunscreen with a sun protection factor (SPF) of 30+, making sure you reapply it every two hours.

Most skin cancers are due to skin damage caused by over-exposure to UV radiation. According to the Australian Cancer Council[8], Australia has one of the highest skin cancer rates in the world. Individuals with skin at higher risk of sun exposure problems tend to burn rather than tan, have naturally red or blonde hair, pale coloured, blue/green eyes and often have freckles. Regular skin checks are advised if you have a personal or family history of skin cancers.

Restorative sleep

Regular restorative sleep is essential for our body to be able to carry out many important housekeeping functions. That includes allowing our skin to recuperate from the environmental assaults of the day. Sleep helps our skin to recover from the redness and damage caused by UV rays and allows DNA repair to reduce the effects of ageing due to sun exposure[9]. The Australian Sleep Foundation[10] recommends that adults 18 to 64 years old aim for between seven to nine hours of uninterrupted sleep each night. Although perimenopause and menopausal hot flushes and night sweats can prove a challenge in getting a decent amount of shut-eye, we can make choices about our bedtime habits, such as ensuring we get to bed on time. You can read more about sleep in the chapter on insomnia.

Smoking

Smoking prematurely ages skin with facial furrows and wrinkles, crows' feet around the eyes and smokers' lines around the lips. It has been said that the skin of a 40-year-old heavy smoker[11] is similar to the skin of a 70-year-old non-smoker[12]. Tobacco-smoking accelerates ageing with its triple whammy effect of decreasing our normal collagen production, increasing the production of matrix metalloproteinase (MMP) which actively breaks down collagen and elastic fibres, and producing reactive oxygen species. Reactive oxygen species are dangerous oxygen molecules that you may have heard being called free radicals. These damage normal skin by causing a cross-linking of collagen and elastin, a process that adds to our wrinkles.

Alcohol

The jury is still out on the effects of alcohol on accelerating skin ageing. A large multiracial study[13] involving participants from Australia, UK, US and Canada reported that drinking eight or more alcoholic drinks per week was associated with more extensive signs of facial aging compared with drinking up to seven alcoholic beverages per week. If you are concerned about the effects of alcohol on your skin, avoid or limit your alcohol intake.

Hydration

Drink enough water. A study[14] found that drinking around eight glasses of water each day will hydrate the deep and superficial layers of the skin. Whilst water is the best hydration option as it contains no calories, other beverages including tea (black, green, and herbal), juice and milk, and vegetables and fruit with high water contents also count toward our daily water intake. Each person's water intake requirements may vary depending on how much exercise or exertion they do, how much they sweat, or on the ambient temperature.

Avoid hot showers and long baths. It is best to avoid hot showers or long, hot baths (get out before your skin starts to look like a prune). Be gentle as you pat yourself dry rather than vigorous rubbing with the towel to avoid damaging your skin's protective barrier.

Moisturise. If you want to reduce moisture loss and skin flaking, it is more effective to apply moisturiser immediately after showering while moisture is still on your skin. Choose a fragrance-free moisturiser to avoid any possible skin sensitivities. There are three broad types of moisturisers: emollient, humectant and occlusive.

Emollient moisturisers. Aging tends to deplete the skin's natural oils and perimenopausal and menopausal women find that emollient moisturisers soothe, smooth and improve skin softness by filling in the small spaces between skin cells on the surface of the skin. If you have dry, irritated or itchy skin that tends to feel worse with soaps, consider using a wash-off emollient as a soap substitute in your tepid to warm but not hot shower. Moisturisers with emollient properties often contain a long list of ingredients of plant, mineral, animal or petroleum origin. When you look at these product labels, you may be familiar with some common examples such as jojoba oil, shea butter, cocoa butter, beeswax, lanolin and petrolatum.

Humectant moisturisers attract water into the surface stratum corneum layer of the skin, hydrating skin by pulling moisture from the air and drawing water from the dermis. However, humectants can be a double-edged sword as the water can easily evaporate and why it is best combined with an occlusive moisturiser (which I will talk about next). Some examples of humectants include honey, sorbitol, glycerine, urea, aloe vera gel, Hyaluronic acid, and Alpha-hydroxy acids such as glycolic acid and lactic acid. Alpha-hydroxy acids (AHAs) are commonly used in anti-ageing skin care products.[15]

Occlusive moisturisers trap and seal in moisture by forming a physical barrier and prevent water loss by evaporation from the deeper epidermis and dermis, and are often combined with humectants. Perimenopausal and menopausal skin may benefit from vegetable or mineral based products.

Vegan-friendly vegetable oils such as grapeseed, coconut, avocado, macadamia, soybean and castor oil are a few examples. Mineral-based petrolatum like Vaseline Intensive Care has an immediate skin-barrier repairing effect[16] and is probably one of the most effective occlusive agents as it prevents 98 per cent of water evaporation though the epidermis[17], though many people find it a bit greasy.

One of the most effective ways to apply moisturiser is to rub it into the palms of your hands first, before lightly applying it to damp skin following a shower or bath.

Jo, I hope you find this helpful.

Yours in good health,

Dr Rosie

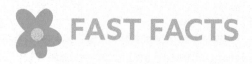

FAST FACTS

Is dryness associated with 'the change' or is it just ageing?

Skin changes occur naturally due to our chronological age, declining oestrogen levels and the influence of our genetics[18]. Our lifestyle choices also influence how dry our skin may appear and feel, such as the years we have spent in the sun, whether or not we smoke, whether or not we drink alcohol, how much sleep we are getting and our exposure to environmental pollution.

Oestrogen is involved in the production of collagen, an important protein building block that helps support our skin and, together with elastic fibres consisting of the protein elastin, serves to maintain the skin's structure and elasticity. Oestrogen also plays a role in the production of natural oils and water-loving glycosaminoglycans (GAGs) that nourish our skin and help retain moisture. Therefore, as hormonal oestrogen declines along with natural oils and the levels of moisture in our skin gets lower, we might find that our skin feels thinner, drier, itchy, flaky and sensitive.

Why can it sometimes feel like there are ants crawling under my skin?

This is a distressing sensation of ants crawling under the skin. In medical-speak this is called *formication*, from the Latin word for ant, *formica*. Some women describe it as more of a tingling, pricking sensation a bit like 'pins and needles'. Lower oestrogen levels can be associated with this sensation.

Is there anything else I can do to look after my skin?

- Use sunscreen and protective clothing
- Stop smoking
- Get a good night's sleep
- Avoid or limit alcohol intake
- Stay well hydrated
- Avoid hot showers and long baths
- Moisturise your skin

Chapter 6
HOT FLUSHES

Global warming

Today I woke up to find my body had caught on fire! Have I arrived – is this my global warming?

Considering I'm not generally one to perspire even with serious athletic exertion, my body presented as if I had just run a marathon. This was a very unusual sensation, to be lying completely still in a ball of sweat at 1:17 a.m. Why had I completely overheated? I had most certainly not undertaken any sexual activity and was pretty sure I wasn't dreaming. I was alone and it was winter.

As I lay still, beads of perspiration formed on my upper lip and my hair was completely saturated. As the sweat found its way down the back of my neck, it gave me the shivers. My torso was clammy, and my legs felt like when I spent a day on the beach as a teenager.

My girlfriends talk about 'hot flushes' and how the sensation of heat builds from their feet to the tip of their head. Parts of their face, neck, and chest start glowing red hot, and beads of sweat add far more than a delicate glow ... some of us are dripping! It takes them completely by surprise, without warning (or even *warning* – cool to scorching in 0.5 seconds!) and often at the most inappropriate times. Actually, when I think of it, 'hot flushes' are unpredictable.

I've heard of various friends complaining about having to change their sleeping environments: overhead fans, air-conditioning, cotton summer sheets (and nothing much else covering hot skin) all year round. With no extra body heat required, the art of spooning has long gone.

Is this our version of global warming – a slow and steady rise in the body's surface temperature, causing thermal expansion (change in body shape) and melting of one's outer crust (make-up)? It sounds relatable but also very depressing. We know actual global warming is having a long-term effect on the earth, and it will be on us if we don't take charge!

Drastic times call for drastic measures. Personal global warming is here and it's changing the look of my wardrobe, whether I like it or not! Farewell polyester and nylon – you are no longer a girl's best friend!

When it's time to hit the streets, cool, breathable, non-hugging, light-weight fabrics appear to be the fashion of choice with many choosing the layered-linen look, which provides the mystery of 'what's lurking beneath the surface'. As you heat you peel, as you cool you layer; it makes perfect sense. But linen creases and therefore is not a sensible attire option in my line of business, and I have no plans of rocking a kaftan in the boardroom anytime soon.

Is it about tricks and illusions, and can we still flaunt it if we're hiding it all away? Thank goodness for the currently soft, floaty fashions that work for those formal occasions. But they too come with their own set of challenges, such as emphasising that feeling of being rounder, thicker and shorter.

Overall, I can't help but notice this personal global warming phenomenon is creating some very poor styling decisions: horizontal stripes across the middle emphasising the MTD (middle-tyre disease).

Is this global warming also the reason why so many midlife women are getting their locks lopped and opting for the stylish short cuts?

I recall a girlfriend telling me that long hair wasn't attractive as we age. I was in my early forties at the time. It was a time to consult my hairdresser, who believes women change their hairstyles for many reasons as they mature. For some, she says, it's a cultural expectation to have their hair cut short as they age. She adds: "Hair is a very important part of a woman's femininity and I encourage women of all ages to keep length in their hair if they choose. Maybe not as long as they wore it as an adolescent but well-maintained, styled long hair comes with a sense of youthfulness, carefree and fun. Elle McPherson, Nicole Kidman and Kylie Minogue are in their fifties and still sporting their golden locks."

Hair at any length *should* make a woman feel beautiful, she says. But another common reason many women forgo long hair after 40 is the heat: to be more comfortable and cooler. Where you live also plays a big part. "Warmer, subtropical climates make shorter hair attractive because it's easy to maintain, whilst in cooler climates long hair is more attractive, for warmth. Women who follow trends will more often than not be the ones showcasing current hairstyles."

It's time to get creative with updos, girls, for those of us who plan on retaining our long hair, although I'm not suggesting the twin plaits are back in fashion – well, not today.

Some of us are having issues with thinning hair, and the battle between the idea of greying with dignity and retaining colour with dyes, including the investment of time and funds, is a topic endlessly debated over coffee and wine.

Thanks to the Japanese who invented the folding fan! Mine are now my newest best friends. I have one each in my car, handbag, work bag, desk, sports bag, yoga bag, by my bedside – everywhere in easy reach. One of my friends who had witnessed my struggles in yoga recently presented me with a hand-held motorised fan; a friend in need is a friend indeed.

So while we struggle with global warming, let's try to do less, wear less and be kinder to ourselves. Let's put more emphasis on our accessories: jewellery, shoes, boots, shawls, scarves, and handbags. I have been told the bigger the handbag, the smaller the arse, if this helps!

Dear Dr Rosie

- What exactly are hot flushes? What causes them?
- Why am I having hot flushes if I'm still in perimenopause, and not yet menopausal?
- Why do some women experience hot flushes and others don't?
- What can I do to prevent or help my hot flushes?

Thanks,
Jo

Let's talk about hot flushes

You've asked some quite specific questions, so let me try to answer them by exploring this topic of hot flushes systematically. Some people call them hot flushes, while others call them hot flashes, and both are correct. So, let's start at the beginning ...

What are hot flushes?

A hot flush is a sudden feeling of heat that spreads over the face, neck, chest and back and may be accompanied by a red flushed face and sweating. Hot flushes can range from mild, described as a transient facial warmth like a blush of embarrassment, to the more severe 'feel-like-I-am-combusting' type, described as a prickly heat that burns in your chest, spreads in a fiery surge upwards into your neck, your face, your forehead, with sweat drenching your hair at the nape of your neck. This is when women tend to break out the fan and ice pack. A severe hot flush can be so disruptive that it makes you stop in your tracks and are unable to continue whatever you were doing. Some women tell me they can also feel shaky, dizzy, headachy or even nauseous and others talk about how they feel anxious and their heart starts pounding. Hot flushes and sweats that happen at night are called night sweats and can contribute to disrupted sleep[1].

Perhaps one of the first things to understand is that not every woman is going to experience hot flushes. In fact, I have consulted with women who were not even sure if they had gone through menopause because they had not been on that often-talked-about rollercoaster ride of on-again, off-again hot flushes. These individuals join two out of ten women who breeze though these transitioning years and pass into menopause without breaking into much of a sweat. However, not every woman who has hot flushes is going to be bothered by them, and generally only about one in five women who are distressed by the discomfort of their hot flushes seek help in treating them[2]. When 152 women in the US were asked to track the severity of their hot flushes and how much they were bothered by their symptoms, 41.3 per cent reported their hot flush symptoms as mild, 43.7 per cent as moderate, 13.1 per cent as severe and 1.8 per cent as very severe[3].

What causes hot flushes?

Although we do not know the exact reason for hot flushes, the latest scientific evidence seems to suggest that sudden changes in oestrogen levels are associated with the onset of hot flushes. Decreased levels of oestrogen cause the thermostat in our brain (the *Star Trek*–sounding 'thermoneutral zone'[4]) to become more sensitive to slight changes in temperature. The brain's thermostat has an upper set point, above which we start to sweat, and a lower set point, below which we get too cold and start to shiver. With a narrower set point, it doesn't take much of a change in core body temperature to trigger a hot flush and/or sweat.

Whilst changing hormonal levels and eventual oestrogen decline appear to play a fundamental role in hot flushes, recent scientific data suggests changing levels of serotonin[5] and norepinephrine (noradrenaline) can also disturb your internal thermostat, which is why some non-hormonal medications like antidepressants, and specifically the serotonin reuptake inhibitors (SSRIs) and serotonin noradrenaline reuptake inhibitors (SNRIs), can help to reduce the distress of hot flushes[6].

In medical-speak, hot flushes and sweats are classified as vasomotor symptoms. That basically means that as your core body temperature rises, the blood vessels just under your skin dilate so that more blood flows to the smaller capillaries and you lose more heat. A hot flush may be accompanied by redness in the face and neck, and you may feel sweaty. As you sweat, the water in the sweat evaporates on your skin and this has a cooling effect. As the hot flush dissipates and the sweat's cooling effect kicks in, your core body temperature goes down, those surface blood vessels respond by constricting and then you can start to shiver as you have hit the lower set point.

And sometimes there can be other reasons for hot flushes. For example, hot flushes share many symptoms with either a high (hyperthyroid) or low (hypothyroid) functioning thyroid (as listed in the following table). If your GP suspects your hot flushes are connected to a thyroid condition or any other reason, this can be checked with a blood test[7].

Hot flushes and symptoms that may be associated with thyroid dysfunction

MENOPAUSE	HYPERTHYROID	HYPOTHYROID
● Hot flushes	● Hot sweats	● Disrupted sleep
● Night sweats	● Anxiety	● Fatigue
● Rapid heart rate	● Rapid heart rate	● Mood swings
● Palpitations	● Weight loss	● Forgetfulness
● Insomnia	● Insomnia	● Depression
● Fatigue		● Irregular periods
● Mood swings		● Weight gain
		● Cold intolerance

How long do hot flushes last?

For the majority of women, those heat surges usually last from one to five minutes. However, there are women whose hot flushes keep going for fifteen minutes. Very occasionally, a hot flush can last for up to one hour.

Hot flushes and night sweats usually last for around five to six years; however, there is a proportion of women who continue to have symptoms for longer than anticipated. The US Penn Ovarian Study[8] looked at individuals who went through a natural menopause and found that about one-third of the participants continued to be bothered by moderately severe hot flushes into their sixties, and around 8 per cent reported that their hot flushes persisted for 20 years.

Why am I having hot flushes if I am still in perimenopause (and not yet menopausal)?

Although we tend to think of ovarian oestrogen as a sex hormone which is limited to working in the reproductive area, the fact of the matter is that oestrogen works in many different areas all over the body. Oestrogen is like a key that will fit and open oestrogen receptor 'locks' in many different parts of the body, and switch on the body's ignition in those particular areas so they can function in the way they are meant to function. We find oestrogen receptors in the breast, brain, bladder, uterus, bones and muscles.

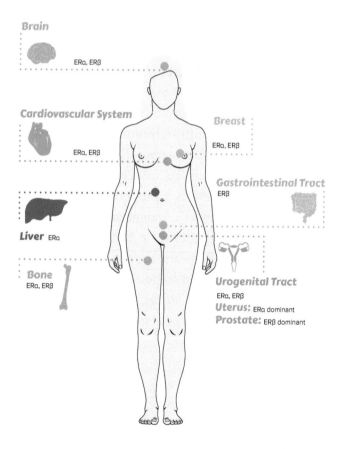

Brain
ERα, ERβ

Cardiovascular System
ERα, ERβ

Breast
ERα, ERβ

Gastrointestinal Tract
ERβ

Liver ERα

Bone
ERα, ERβ

Urogenital Tract
ERα, ERβ
Uterus: ERα dominant
Prostate: ERβ dominant

During the perimenopausal transition, as oestrogen levels fluctuate and eventually start declining, the effects of lower oestrogen levels will also be experienced in other parts of the body. It is important to understand that during a natural perimenopause transition, although oestrogen levels decline, they do not stop abruptly or fall to zero[9]. Lower oestrogen levels in the bladder may cause symptoms of needing to urinate more frequently. Lower levels of oestrogen working in the brain may reset the set-points of our internal temperature-regulating system and we may experience hot flushes. Lower levels of oestrogen working on oestrogen receptors in the skin can be experienced as dry skin. In other words, wherever oestrogen receptors are located and there is decreased oestrogen activity, we may experience symptoms including:

- hot flushes, sweating, night sweats (see chapters 7 & 8)
- heart discomfort, such as having an awareness of heartbeats, palpitations, a racing heart (see chapter 4)
- sleep disruptions, such as difficulty falling asleep, staying asleep and/or early-morning waking (see chapter 9)
- mood swings, feelings of sadness, depressed mood, a lack of motivation (see chapter 4)
- irritability, feelings of inner tension or aggressiveness (see chapter 4)
- anxiety, such as feeling panicky or restless (see chapter 4)
- physical and mental fatigue, decreased concentration, forgetfulness
- sexual issues, such as changes in sexual desire, libido, activity and satisfaction (see chapter 11)
- bladder problems, such as needing to urinate more

frequently and/or urgently, bladder incontinence (see chapter 12)

* vaginal dryness, a feeling of burning or dryness, difficulty with intercourse (see chapter 10)
* muscular aches and pains.

I'd like you to understand that the way one woman experiences the effects of declining oestrogen levels may be different from the way another woman experiences those perimenopausal changes. This transition to menopause is going to be different for each woman because each woman is more than simply the sum of her hormones. Changing hormone levels are only one piece of a much larger puzzle that makes you uniquely you.

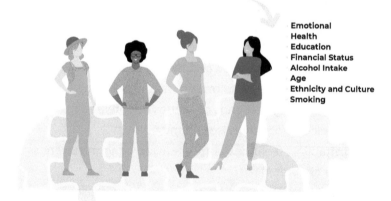

CHANGING HORMONE LEVELS ARE ONLY ONE PIECE OF THE PUZZLE

Emotional
Health
Education
Financial Status
Alcohol Intake
Age
Ethnicity and Culture
Smoking

Why do some women experience hot flushes and others don't?

During the transition from perimenopause through menopause, up to eight out of every ten women in Australia are likely to experience hot flushes. Individuals who smoke, are an unhealthy weight or lead a sedentary lifestyle have been found to have a greater tendency to experience hot flushes.

What can I do to help myself?

Most women find that if their hot flushes are mild, some simple lifestyle changes may be enough to cope with their symptoms. Many women find that making some lifestyle changes to control their environment and avoid triggers that lead to overheating is the easiest way to manage mild to moderate hot flushes.

Dress in layers. Layering in linen or other natural fibres like cotton allows your skin to breathe. I have gotten into the habit of always carrying an oversized wrap shawl in my bag to cover up, whether I'm travelling or sitting in the cinema. A wrap doesn't have to break the bank and can add that splash of colour to a neutral outfit. Funnily enough, I have received many more compliments for a couple of wraps that cost me $20 than for other expensive items.

Keep it cool. Carrying a fan and water small spray-bottle of water in your handbag or backpack is helpful. Working in an air-conditioned office is a plus for many women. Keep your bedroom cool with fan(s) or air-conditioning and use breathable sheets. Tuck a cold pack into your pillow and turn your pillow over when it starts to feel hot.

Control your caffeine intake. You might find it helpful to avoid or reduce your intake of caffeine. OK, OK – that heart-starter coffee in the morning may be non-negotiable and that is OK. For some women, even one cup of coffee is too much, however, and if you are consuming three to four cups a day then perhaps it's time to reflect on why. If you need caffeine to keep you moving and focused, then re-evaluate how much you are demanding of yourself. If, on the other hand, it is simply a matter of taste and choice, then consider decreasing the amount you drink or changing to decaf. Some people can go cold turkey and give up coffee in one hit. But if you decide to cut down on caffeine abruptly, you may end up with a massive headache. Therefore, consider reducing your coffee intake by a cup every few days in a gradual weaning process and reducing the strength from full strength to half strength. And remember some teas, cola and energy drinks and hot chocolate are caffeinated too. The other factor to think about is whether it might be the temperature of the beverage that is problematic for you; some women find that the hotness of the drink is what tends to trigger a hot flush, so cool drinks are the way to go.

Avoid spicy foods. Avoiding spicy foods may or may not make a difference to your hot flushes. If curries and Thai food make you perspire, they are best avoided. Having said that, it is always a personal choice. For example, you may be out shopping one day and decide not to gather the ingredients to make that curry you saw a recipe for, whereas another time you may be with family and friends in 'social celebration' mode at a restaurant and decide to just enjoy the food, hot flushes be damned. Some women feel empowered by taking an 80:20 approach, which means they will avoid spicy foods most of the time but when they want to indulge, it is their conscious choice to do so.

Stay hydrated. It is essential that you ensure that you drink plenty of water to maintain hydration because when we sweat, water evaporates, and the thirst signal does not accurately reflect how hydrated we are. A really simple way to know if you are drinking enough water is to check the colour of your urine, which should be very pale yellow. If your urine is darker than a pale-straw colour, then you are not drinking enough water.

So, what can you do to help yourself if you have been careful to avoid hot-flush triggers and made changes to your environment but are still suffering with moderate to severe symptoms? You may consider these options:

- hormonal medications
- bioidentical hormones
- non-hormonal medications
- complementary and alternative medicine (CAM).

We will look at these more closely in the next two chapters.

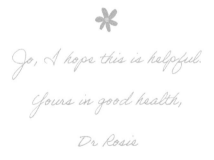

Jo, I hope this is helpful.

Yours in good health,

Dr Rosie

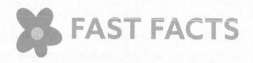 # FAST FACTS

What are hot flushes?

A hot flush is a sudden feeling of heat that spreads over the face, neck, chest and back and may be accompanied by a red flushed face and sweating. Hot flushes and sweats that happen at night are called night sweats and can contribute to disrupted sleep.

What causes hot flushes?

Although we do not know the exact reason for hot flushes, the latest scientific evidence seems to suggest that sudden changes in oestrogen levels are associated with the onset of hot flushes. Decreased levels of oestrogen cause the thermostat in our brain to become more sensitive to slight changes in temperature. With a narrower set point, it doesn't take much of a change in core body temperature to trigger a hot flush and/or sweat. Recent scientific information also suggests changing levels of serotonin and norepinephrine (noradrenaline) can also disturb your internal thermostat.

How long do hot flush last?

For the majority of women, those heat surges usually last from one to five minutes. However, there are women whose hot flushes keep going for fifteen minutes. Very occasionally, a hot flush can last for up to one hour.

Hot flushes and night sweats usually last for around five to six years.

The large US Penn Ovarian study which looked at women who experienced a natural menopause, found that about onethird of women continued to be bothered by moderately severe hot flushes into their sixties, and around 8 per cent reported that their hot flushes persisted for 20 years.

Why do some women experience hot flushes and others don't?

That is a very good question and one that researchers are still trying to answer. What we do know is that two out of ten women transition into menopause without breaking into much of a sweat. Individuals who smoke, are an unhealthy weight or lead a sedentary lifestyle have been found to have a greater tendency to experience hot flushes.

What can I do to help myself?
Control your environment

- Dress in layers of natural cotton or linen fabrics that allow your skin to breathe.
- Carry a fan and water spray-bottle in your handbag.
- Working in an air-conditioned office is a plus for many women.
- Keep your bedroom cool with fan(s) or air-conditioning.
- Tuck a cold pack into your pillow and turn your pillow over when it starts to feel hot.

Avoid hot flush triggers

- Avoid or reduce your intake of caffeine and spicy foods.
- Consider avoiding or reducing alcohol if this triggers a hot flush – find out what works best for you.

* Drink plenty of water to maintain hydration.

If you have already been avoiding hot flush triggers and making changes to your environment but are still suffering with symptoms, then there are other options:

* hormonal medications
* bioidentical hormones
* non-hormonal medications
* complementary and alternative medicine (CAM).

Chapter 7
HORMONE THERAPY

To HRT or not to HRT – that is the question

Hormone replacement therapy is a thought-provoking phrase; it's a battle I have with myself and a controversial discussion I have with others: should or shouldn't we do HRT?

"Oh no, not now," I thought as I felt the heat build on my face and my scalp began to perspire.

Generally, I would only experience this sensation after I had eaten chillies or a hot Indian curry. This was not a good time, especially in the middle of presenting to a new client for business in their home. As I tried my hardest to contain myself and remain focused, I could feel the sweat travelling from the nape of my neck, down my spine, along the backs of my legs to my ankles. My shoes filling with water and my feet feeling squishy took me back to my childhood memories of walking home in sodden school shoes in a Melbourne winter. My focus had quickly changed and my brain was awash; I felt severe brain fog, similar to 'baby brain'; my concentration now lost. Sweat continued to roll down my torso, sending a shiver up my spine, and I realised I was completely plastered to the upholstery of the seat. I was thankful I had made the decision to wear a black dress that day. I needed to remain as still as possible to avoid sounding like wet washing sloshing around inside a washing machine. At that moment, I was quite a sight: with my flushing face, drenched head of hair perfectly stuck to my head and the sleek new sheen my dress had acquired.

There was no coming back from this debacle. I hoped that my episode had slipped under the radar and gone undetected until my client began opening every window and turning on every fan to full capacity. As I stood to 'exit stage left', I was afraid of looking down out of fear that I had created two puddles from where my feet were planted.

Ironically, my sister shares a very similar story of our mother during an 'offertory procession' at church, where she dripped all the way down the aisle in squelching shoes and a face as red as a beetroot.

Enough was enough, and it was at that moment when I walked back to my car that I decided I could not continue to work under these conditions. My natural therapies had failed me, and it was time for a new approach.

I know very little about hormone replacement therapy. My fear is provoked by my lack of knowledge. Hormone replacement therapy – the words alone scare me, suggesting artificial hormones, breast and ovarian cancers, a third breast growing on my back and an extra 20 kilos!

Those of us who have experienced pregnancy tend to have a birth plan in mind prior to labour which may include little to no pain relief. But, to our surprise, once we're actually in labour, we beg for gas, an epidural and/or a caesarean – anything that will dull the pain, alleviate the stress and allow us to deliver quickly and safely.

I'm almost certain that one shoe does not fit most, but as I sit in my living room with my girlfriends discussing HRT, we are divided. Two out of five would consider HRT and the remaining three are adamant that they would never take artificial hormones. Surprisingly, the two women for (including me) are right in the midst of debilitating perimenopause symptoms, whilst the three younger women against are not there yet. If they were, I wonder if they would have a different opinion?

It's comforting to know that help is at hand and we don't need to struggle or suffer. We have a choice to decide if HRT is right for us or not, and that is the true beauty!

Well, Dr Rosie, these are my questions for you.

- What is hormone replacement therapy?
- Is it safe?
- How long do you remain on HRT?
- How effective is HRT?
- Are there any alternatives to HRT?

Thanks,
Jo

Let's talk about HRT

Dear Jo,

Thank you for your questions. My first recommendation here is to book a long appointment with your doctor to have a conversation that relates to your particular circumstances, because any recommendations are going to be on a case-by-case basis. Any discussions about hormones require a comprehensive appointment in which your doctor is going to be asking you a lot of questions about your current and past medical history including cervical and breast health screening. You're going to have a physical examination which will include blood pressure, weight and attending to any screening issues if required. When we talk about HRT, the main reason a woman may consider using it is to relieve symptoms of moderate to severe hot flushes and night sweats, when distressing and frequent.

Imagine addressing a meeting red faced, dripping sweat, squelching in your shoes with a feeling of brain fog and having difficulty with finding the right words. For those women who are really suffering, hormone replacement can have a dramatic difference in relieving their symptoms and improving their ability to function.

What is hormone replacement therapy?

Hormone replacement therapy (HRT) is the name used for medications that contain hormones used to treat bothersome menopausal symptoms of hot flushes, night sweats and vaginal dryness. Another name you may see being used is menopause replacement therapy (MRT). The name change reflects the recent changes in hormone formulations that have made them more closely resemble the natural hormones our body makes. However, I am going to use HRT because most people are familiar with that terminology.

HRT is based on oestrogen and progesterone to mimic the effects of the hormones our body naturally makes. The formulations include:

* oestrogen with progestogen. You will often see the word progestogen used, an umbrella term to cover both natural progesterone your body makes and the synthetic form.
* oestrogen only – used for those who have had a hysterectomy as the protective effect of progesterone against the build-up of the uterus (womb) lining is no longer required.
* progesterone only.

HRT is available in a number of ways:

* oral tablets
* gels or transdermal patches as hormones can be absorbed through the skin
* creams or pessaries – dissolvable tablets that can be inserted into the vagina.

HRT is like a bridge to help your body adjust to lower levels of oestrogen +/- progesterone that occur with menopause. Whilst you take HRT, the medication is doing the work. The good news is that although women's naturally made ovarian oestrogen (oestradiol) levels significantly decrease by the time women reach menopause, they do not drop to zero because the body adapts and makes weaker forms of oestrogen (namely oestrone) in other parts of the body[1] (see chapter one).

The amount of oestrogen used for HRT in menopause is typically lower than the amount that a combined hormonal contraceptive pill taken by perimenopausal women during their reproductive years contains, which is why it is unsuitable for contraceptive coverage[2].

How effective is hormone therapy in managing my distressing symptoms?

Hormone therapy has been shown to be the most effective treatment for hot flushes, night sweats, vaginal dryness and in the prevention of fractures and bone loss. The most effective treatment for managing hot flushes is oestrogen, either alone or combined with progestogen, with a reported 75 percent reduction in weekly hot flash frequency and reduction in severity compared to placebo[3].

Although effective, HRT is not going to be medically suitable for everyone. When you sit down with your doctor, you will be assessed to find out if you have certain conditions when HRT is contraindicated (not safe) and your needs will be determined on a case-by-case basis. Conditions, when a transdermal patch, gel or cream is prescribed, that may be OK include cardiovascular disease, current or previous blood clots, liver disease and possibly migraine with aura.

If you are suffering with distressing symptoms and unable or prefer not to take HRT, there are other options available that we will look at in another chapter.

To HRT or not to HRT? That indeed is the question

First, let's look at the 'not to HRT'. We have already noted that there are many women for whom hormone therapy is not a safe option, because they have medically recognised conditions that would increase their risk of developing breast cancer, blood clots, heart disease and stroke. There are also many women who would not consider HRT, who prefer to do things naturally and want nothing to do with prescribed hormones, who are concerned about the safety of conventional hormone therapy and mistrust a medical system they see as heavily reliant on prescribing medication. I'll tell you a bit more about complementary and non-hormonal options that women might choose in the next chapter.

Let's move on the 'to HRT' part.

Is HRT safe?

If you have been furiously fanning yourself at your desk or dripping in boardroom meetings, relieving those bothersome, embarrassing hot flushes and soaking sweats can make a difference in your ability to cope day to day. If you have found that lifestyle measures or other therapies have helped a bit but are not enough to manage your distressing symptoms, then HRT is highly effective as a treatment. Whilst the benefits of HRT include its effectiveness in relieving symptoms and improving your quality of life, as with any medication, there are some risks to consider. What I have found is that woman considering HRT tend to worry about the big C, which is the risk of breast cancer and that is understandable as breast cancer is the most common cancer affecting Australian women. To better understand where this concern has come from and put it into perspective, let's take a quick trip down HRT memory lane.

In the early 20th century, menopausal symptoms like hot flushes and vaginal dryness were considered an 'hormonal deficiency syndrome'[4]. In 1942, Premarin, made from pregnant horse urine, was the first approved HRT medication. In the 1960s, a gynaecologist, Robert A. Wilson advised that taking oestrogen pills to correct the oestrogen deficiency would maintain a woman's femininity, "breasts and genital organs will not shrivel. She will be much more pleasant to live with and will not become dull and unattractive."

For decades, women hot and bothered by hot flushes and night sweats found that oestrogen effectively reduced the frequency of hot flushes by up to 75 percent[5]. Oestrogen also has a protective effect on heart and blood vessels but in the ten years after starting menopause, with a significant decrease in oestrogen levels, the risk of heart attack and stroke in women increases. Over the years, researchers had observed HRT and its effect on women's health in a number of studies like the Nurses' Health Study[6] and the Million Women Study[7]. The question was posed: could HRT be used to prevent major age-related diseases such as cardiovascular disease in post-menopausal women?

The 1990s US Women's Health Initiative[8] (WHI) study put this question to the test. This large clinical trial involved more than 160,000 healthy women aged 50 to 79. Participants were randomly assigned to one of three trial groups. One group, women with a uterus, were started on PremPro (oestrogen and progestogen, a synthetic progesterone, combination), another group who had undergone hysterectomy used oestrogen only, and the third group were given a placebo (no active ingredient).

In 2002, the oestrogen and progestogen part of the trial was stopped three years earlier than planned, as the results showed an increase in breast cancer, heart disease, stroke and blood clots. Although results had shown a reduction in the risk of colon cancer and bone fractures, it was widely publicised in the media that the risks of HRT outweighed the benefits. After the WHI reported these findings, an unprecedented number of women all over the world stopped using their HRT. With the sudden cessation of HRT use, many women had a return of their previously debilitating symptoms.

When the WHI study was later re-examined[9], there was a lot of discussion about the age at which the hormone treatments were started and the way in which the results were reported. The average age of participants in the WHI study was 63, which is at least ten years later than HRT is normally started. Questions were raised on whether the age at which women were commenced on HRT makes a different to their risks. Re-examination of the WHI data found that the risk of breast cancer for women on the oestrogen plus progestogen increased risk with the age at which their HRT was started.

The types of oestrogen and progesterone preparations used in those studies are now more than twenty years old. The WHI hormones are like comparing a mobile phone from the 1990s, which was more like a brick, to the streamlined mobiles of today. There are HRT preparations used today which are identical to the oestrogen (E2) made by your ovaries and a body identical progesterone derived from wild Mexican yams which is the same formulation your ovaries make.

The current understanding of the data reports the absolute risk of breast cancer for a woman using oestrogen and progestogen, on average is less than one women per 1000 in 12 months.

You may be wondering if there are other factors that increase the likelihood of developing breast cancer. There is no getting away from it: being female and increasing age are two risk factors for breast cancer. A family history of breast cancer, age at menarche when you get your first period, age of first birth, and experiencing a late menopause after the age of 55 are also factors associated with later-life breast cancer. Many people are unaware that being an unhealthy weight (BMI > 25kg/m2) and drinking at two alcoholic drinks per day increase your risk of breast cancer compared to HRT users.

Being breast aware is something you can do. A good place to get to know your breasts is in the shower because when you know what is normal for your breasts, you will recognise if there are any unusual changes in your breasts.

Breast changes to watch for include:

- a new lump or any lumpiness, especially if it is only in one breast
- change in size or shape of the breast
- dimpling or redness of breast skin
- nipple redness, crusting, discharge, ulcer, inversion (there is a change in the nipple so it pulls inwards)
- breast pain that does not go away.

Not all breast changes are due to cancer however; it is very important to visit you GP without delay and have any concerns checked out, even if you have had a recent normal mammogram.

In Australia, women who are aged 50–74 without any symptoms can have a free screening with BreastScreen every two years. However, screening is available for women aged 40-49 which can be discussed with your doctor. I would like to emphasise that if you notice any changes or have concerns, please visit your GP sooner rather than later, and have it checked out.

The benefits of HRT include a reduction in distressing symptoms such as hot flushes, night sweats, vaginal dryness and urinary symptoms, improved quality of life, and a reduction in the risk of developing osteoporosis, cardiovascular and colorectal cancer. When my patients are weighing up the benefits and risks about HRT, I often suggest they 'think like a judge'. When you think like a judge you would look at the evidence that answers: What are the benefits? How effective is this particular option in managing or reducing my distressing and debilitating symptom(s)?

The issue of safety is important so you would consider: What are **the risks**? Are there any **negative side effects**?

Then place your answers on the scales and weigh up each side, and consider how **important** the benefits and risks are for you.

I suggest that when you think like a judge, you can apply these questions impartially to any lifestyle change, medication, supplement or therapy you are considering.

The concerns regarding HRT and increased health risks of breast cancer and heart disease continue to be controversial and a source of ongoing discussion and research. If you are considering HRT, remember to book that long appointment long appointment with your doctor as you can now understand, each person needs to be assessed on an individual basis and there is a lot to discuss.

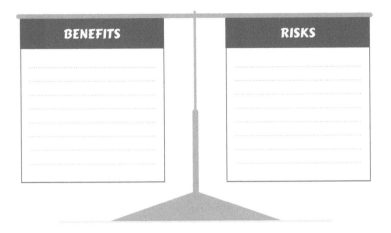

When to start HRT?

According to the International Menopause Society, HRT is best started before the age of 60 in women with moderate to severe symptoms who do not have any contraindications[xcix]. Generally, in a woman suffering with distressing symptoms who is under the age of 60 or it is less than 10 years since she started menopause, the benefits appear to outweigh the risks for commencing this therapy. There is limited data for continued use of HRT after the age of 60.

How long do I remain on HRT?

Australian and international guidelines recommend that HRT be determined on an individual basis. Doctors usually prescribe HRT at the lowest possible dose for the least amount of time, to effectively relieve distressing symptoms of menopause. It is important that any woman using HRT visit her doctor regularly to monitor her blood pressure, weight, ensure her screening is up to date and review if she can stop taking it as soon as she no longer needs it. When the time comes to stop HRT, it is usually recommended to come off the medication gradually to reduce the likelihood of symptoms returning and many women tend to find timing this process during the cooler months is easier than during the hotter time of year.

Are there any alternatives to HRT?

You mentioned in your letter that you'd already tried some natural therapies, so I'm sure you'll be interested to know about the alternatives for women who can't – or choose not to – undertake HRT. These include bioidentical hormones, non-hormonal medication, and complementary and alternative medicine therapies. I have quite a bit to tell you about them, Jo, so I will send you another letter very soon.

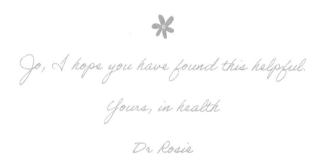

Jo, I hope you have found this helpful.

Yours, in health

Dr Rosie

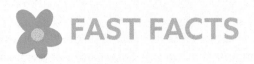 **FAST FACTS**

What is HRT?

Hormone replacement therapy (HRT) is the name used for several medications that contain hormones used to treat menopausal symptoms. Another name you may see used is menopause replacement therapy (MRT). HRT is based on oestrogen and progesterone hormones our body makes and is available in a number of ways:

- oral tablets
- gels or transdermal patches as hormones can be absorbed through the skin
- creams or pessaries – dissolvable tablets that can be inserted into the vagina.

Is HRT effective?

It is reported that systemic oestrogen is the most effective therapy to manage the distressing symptoms of bothersome moderate to severe hot flushes, reported to reduce hot flush frequency by 75 percent, as well as helping with night sweats and sometimes joint pains. Additionally, oestrogen improves bone health to prevent bone loss and fracture.

Is hormone therapy safe?

Current international and Australian guidelines recommend commencing HRT in healthy women 50–59 years who are suffering with moderate to severe symptoms. Although effective, no medication is without risks and therefore every individual needs to be considered on a case-by-case basis. Generally, however, the benefits appear to outweigh the risks for commencing HRT treatment of symptomatic women aged under 60 or less than 10 years since they started menopause. There is limited data on continued use of HRT after the age of 60. The concerns regarding HRT and increased health risks of breast cancer and heart disease continue to be controversial and a source of ongoing discussion and research. If you are considering HRT, I recommend booking a long appointment with your doctor each person needs to be assessed on an individual basis and there is a lot to discuss.

How long do you remain on HRT?

Australian and international guidelines recommend that HRT be used at the lowest possible dose for the least amount of time to effectively relieve distressing symptoms. Many women use HRT for less than five years. It is important that any woman using HRT visit her doctor regularly to monitor blood pressure, weight, ensure screening is up to date and review whether to stop taking HRT as soon as she no longer needs it. When the time comes to stop HRT, it is usually recommended to wean off the medication gradually to reduce the likelihood of symptoms returning.

Some helpful websites and resources:

Jean Hailes for Women's Health
https://www.jeanhailes.org.au/

Australian Menopause Society – website fact sheets:
https://www.menopause.org.au/health-info/fact-sheets

Australian Government Cancer Australia – lifestyle choices to reduce your risk for cancer: https://canceraustralia.gov.au/healthy-living/lifestyle-risk-reduction

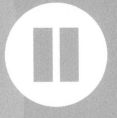

Chapter 8
OTHER THERAPIES

Let's talk about alternate therapies

In my last letter, I promised to write to you about alternative options to HRT, as I'm sure you've got questions about them. Whilst many women have found HRT to be effective for managing their distressing hot flushes, night sweats and vaginal dryness, it is not a treatment that is going to be suitable or acceptable for every individual. There are many women for whom hormone therapy is not a safe option, because they have medically recognised conditions that would increase their risk of developing breast cancer, blood clots, heart disease and stroke.

There are also many women who prefer to do things naturally and want nothing to do with prescribed hormones, who are concerned about the safety of conventional hormone therapy and mistrust a medical system they see as heavily reliant on prescribing medication. In a British online survey[1] of 1464 perimenopausal women, 41 per cent stated they would never take HRT and 77 per cent said they would prefer to use alternative therapies rather than hormone therapy.

So, what are the options for those women who are distressed by their symptoms but are unable to use HRT or prefer not to use this therapy? The options include bioidentical hormones, non-hormonal medications and complementary and alternative therapies.

Bioidentical hormones

Although compounded bioidentical hormones are generally thought of as natural because they are based on plants such as soy or wild yam, they still need to be synthesised in the laboratory, just as many vitamins are synthesised in the lab. Bioidentical hormones are defined by the Endocrine Society as "compounds that have exactly the same chemical and molecular structure as hormones that are produced in the human body"[2]. There is an assumption that compounded bioidentical hormones deliver the same benefits as preparations which are standardised and regulated by the Australian Therapeutics Goods Administration (TGA) but without the potential harms some feel might come with using HRT. The problem with non-TGA-approved compounded hormones is that there is no regulation of production quality, purity, concentration and dosage of the contents with an investigation finding that this can be variable even in the same batch of troches, capsules or cream[3].

A 2016 Cochrane review which pulled evidence together from all the available studies said: "No data are yet available about the safety of bioidentical hormone therapy with regard to long-term outcomes such as heart attack, stroke and breast cancer."[4] It would seem logical that the same risks attributed to HRT be attributed to bioidentical hormones also. At this stage, there have been no studies which demonstrate otherwise.

Nevertheless, you may be surprised to know that there are a number of TGA-approved versions of oestradiol and micronised progesterone identical to the hormones your ovaries make.

Non-hormonal medications

There are several pharmaceutical medications that have been shown to help with reducing the distress of hot flushes and night sweats.

Non-hormonal pharmaceutical medications may be an option for women who experience moderate to severe hot flushes and have had or are at risk of breast or endometrial cancer, blood clots, heart disease or stroke, which may preclude them from using hormonal therapy. They are an option for women who choose not to use HRT and those who have tried natural therapies but have not found them to be helpful in relieving their distressing symptoms. As for any medication, you will need to speak with your doctor as to whether this type of therapy is suitable for you in your situation and consider any negative side effects.

Antidepressants: SSRIs and SNRIs

SSRI stands for selective serotonin reuptake inhibitor; escitalopram, citalopram, and paroxetine are commonly prescribed SSRIs. SNRI stands for serotonin norepinephrine reuptake inhibitor; and an example of an SNRI is venlafaxine (Effexor). These types of antidepressants have been found to be effective in reducing moderate to severe hot flushes as a non-hormonal alternative to hormone therapy. Generally, a trial of four weeks low to moderate doses of these medications is enough time to discover if they are helpful for you. Common side effects include nausea and drowsiness. Some people taking higher doses of venlafaxine[5] experience dry mouth, headache, constipation, nausea and a decrease in appetite.

Escitalopram

In a double-blind randomised control trial of escitalopram (SSRI)[6], a group of women taking either 10 mg/day or 20 mg/day of escitalopram was compared with a group who took a placebo (inactive sugar pill). The researchers were trying to work out how effective the medication was in reducing the severity, frequency and nuisance value of hot flushes as well as how well it is tolerated by women taking the different dosages. After eight weeks of the trial, 55 per cent of the women taking either dose of escitalopram had a 50 per cent decrease in the frequency and severity of their hot flushes compared with 36 per cent in the placebo group.

Safety profile: The medication was well tolerated with no significant side effects reported.

Venlafaxine

Venlafaxine (SNRI)[7] also has been shown to reduce hot flushes. A randomised control trial reported a 37 to 61 per cent reduction in hot flushes after six weeks of treatment starting with 37.5 mg/day for one week and then 75 mg/day.

Safety profile: At higher doses, more side effects were reported and included a dry mouth, headache, constipation, nausea and decreased appetite.

Clonidine

Clonidine is a medication to reduce high blood pressure that was first used as a treatment for hot flushes in the 1970s. Meta-analysis[8] of 10 trials showed inconsistent results with half the studies reporting a reduction of hot flushes by one hot flush per day, and the other studies reporting no significant difference.

Safety profile: Side effects of clonidine include dry mouth, constipation, dizziness, drowsiness and itching. This medication is not used often given the high likelihood of experiencing these side effects and the availability of other, better-tolerated options.

Gabapentin

Gabapentin, an anticonvulsant, has been used to effectively reduce hot flushes and may be particularly useful for managing those night sweats. One study[9] involving 100 healthy post-menopausal women aged 45 to 65 found that gabapentin at 300 mg/day was as effective as oestrogen in reducing the frequency and severity of hot flushes.

Safety profile: Gastrointestinal discomfort may occur at lower doses such as 300 mg/day. Higher doses are associated with drowsiness, dizziness and disorientation.

Complementary and alternative medicine (CAM) therapies

Although menopause is a natural process, for some women, the symptoms can be so distressing that they find them to be disabling. After the release of the Women's Health Initiative (WHI) findings in 2002, there has been much confusion about the benefits and risks associated with hormone treatment. As a result, many midlife women looked for more natural ways to manage their menopausal symptoms and turned to dietary and herbal therapies such as black cohosh, a range of phytoestrogens which are plant-based compounds that mimic the effects of oestrogen and found in soy and isoflavone products, yoga, meditation, massage, aromatherapy and other complementary and alternative (CAM) therapies to relieve their symptoms.

What is meant by CAM therapies?

According to the US National Centre for Complementary and Integrative Medicine, these CAM therapies are "health care approaches that are not typically part of conventional medical care or that may have origins outside of usual Western practices"[10]. Complementary means that the therapy is used together with mainstream medicine, and alternative means the non-mainstream practice is used instead of conventional medicine. CAM therapies can be grouped under three broad categories:

- natural products, such as herbs, vitamins, minerals, and dietary supplements
- mind-body practices, such as hypnosis, meditation, relaxation, aromatherapy, and cognitive behavioural therapy (CBT)
- whole-system approaches which may use a combination of both mind-body practices and natural products, and include acupuncture, Chinese medicine, reflexology and homeopathy.

Natural Products	Mind-Body Practices	Whole System Approaches
Herbs	Hypnosis	Traditional Chinese medicine
Vitamins	Cognitive behavioural therapy (CBT)	Acupuncture
Minerals		Reflexology
Dietary supplements	Yoga	Homeopathy
	Relaxation	
	Meditation	
	Paced breathing	
	Aromatherapy	

When 2020 Australian women aged 40–65 were invited to answer questions about their use of CAM therapies, just under 40 per cent reported they were using CAM therapies to manage their menopausal symptoms, and 13.3 per cent were using this type of therapy specifically for dealing with their hot flushes[11]. In this particular study, the most commonly used CAM therapies used to manage hot flushes were found to be phytoestrogens (plant-based compounds that mimic the effect of oestrogen) and herbal supplements including evening primrose oil, ginseng and black cohosh. Other popular botanical over-the-counter products include red clover, dong quai, and wild yam; all available in several different forms such as teas, tinctures, pills, and creams.

How effective are CAM therapies?

Whilst a large number of women who use CAM believe them to be very helpful, just how effective are these treatments? More than 10,000 women aged 50 to 65 in the UK[12] who had stopped using HRT after the WHI report were asked about the type of CAM therapy they used and whether they found them effective. Whilst the most popular herbal remedies were evening primrose and black cohosh, more women said that they found regular exercise, yoga, counselling and CBT were more helpful and effective compared with the herbal remedies.

When put to the test, a review[13] of a variety of CAM to manage menopausal symptoms found that hypnosis and CBT safe and effective in managing hot flushes, sleep regulation and sexual dysfunction, for example, hypnosis specifically used to manage hot flushes was able to reduce hot flushes by at least 50 per cent. Mindfulness-based stress reduction and relaxation techniques were found to help reduce and manage stress during the perimenopausal transition.

Herbal products and food supplements have been studied for their effectiveness in reducing menopausal symptoms. Black cohosh and soy isoflavones (derived from plants) are two standardised preparations which have been subjected to several high-quality randomised controlled trials and large scientific reviews, and yet, when the results of several studies of the same herb or the same supplement have been examined, reports of effectiveness are often conflicting. For example, in one high-quality trial to see if black cohosh reduced the frequency of hot flushes and improved their quality of life – in other words, participant's level of comfort and satisfaction – there was no difference between the participants using the herb and those individuals who used the placebo[14]. Compare this to another high-quality study in which black cohosh was combined with St John's wort, which concluded the black cohosh combined with St John's wort group was superior to the placebo in reducing distressing menopausal symptoms as associated distress[15]. So why the differences in results?

Although many herbal products are manufactured to a high-quality standard, other products are variable in their purity and level of active ingredients. The large variability in the quality, concentration of active ingredient, dosage, whether herbs are tested on their own or in combination formula, and even the variability in the way in which a study is conducted, and ways in which results are reported can make it difficult when research results are combined. As herbs usually take longer to work compared to HRT, even the duration of a study may be too short to determine benefit. It is a bit like trying to compare apples with oranges. Therefore, it comes as no surprise that authors of large reviews with so many variations usually conclude there is no consistent or convincing evidence that herbal preparations are more effective than placebo.

According to the North American Menopause Society (NAMS), whilst the most effective treatment for managing menopausal symptoms is hormone-based therapy, "CAM approaches, including acupuncture, herbal products, dietary soy and isoflavone products may be offered to treat vasomotor symptoms, although clinical trials generally demonstrate benefit for menopausal symptoms similar to that of placebo."[16]

There are a couple of things to point out from this state-ment. Firstly, clinical trials conducted on these CAM therapies generally demonstrate benefit. In other words, there is *a benefit demonstrated* which is different from a study showing that there is no benefit. The second issue is that the benefit for menopausal symptoms *is similar to that of placebo.*

When the word placebo is mentioned, it is often thought of in a negative way, that any effect is 'all in your head'. You may be surprised to know that the 'placebo effect' is indeed an effect that needs to be accounted for in any high-quality clinical trial. Let's now take a quick peek at what happened when naturally occurring plant-based compounds commonly used to manage hot flushes were put to the test.

Black cohosh (*Cimicifuga racemosa*) has traditionally been used by American Indians for menstrual irregularity and is commonly used by women for troublesome perimenopausal and menopausal symptoms such as hot flushes. The root (or rhizome) of the plant is used and contains several chemically active ingredients. The Australian Menopause Society supports this view but also advises that the effectiveness of black cohosh in improving hot flushes, night sweats and bone health has not yet been established and suggests that further research is required.

Safety profile: The US National Institutes of Health (NIH) reported that the most common negative side effects of black cohosh include gastrointestinal upset, dizziness, headache, nausea, vomiting and rashes[17].

Red clover (*Trifolium pratense*) is a bright pink flowering plant which belongs to the legume (pea) family and traditionally used in North America as a medicinal plant and more recently as a menopausal herb. Red clover contains isoflavones, a type of plant oestrogen (see phytoestrogens below) that produce an oestrogen-like effect. A comprehensive review[18] which looked at five studies using a standardised 80 mg/day extract concluded the group taking red clover demonstrated a significant decrease in the frequency of hot flushes compared to the placebo group.

Phytoestrogens are naturally occurring plant-based compounds with a similar chemical structure to our body's ovarian oestrogen. Phytoestrogens can bind to our oestrogen receptors and weakly mimic the actions of our body's oestrogens.

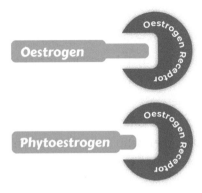

Phytoestrogens are found in over 300 plant species and there are three main classes of phytoestrogens with oestrogenic properties: isoflavones, coumestans and lignins. Some common foods containing these compounds are listed in the table below.

Table of categories of phytoestrogens and common food sources

ISOFLAVONES	COUMESTANS	LIGNINS
Soybeans	Soybeans	Flax/ linseed
Red clover	Red clover	Tea (green & black)
Alfalfa	Alfalfa sprouts	Sunflower seeds
Lentils		Barley
Chickpeas		Hops
Beans		Rye
		Rice
		Oats

Although up to 80 per cent of Western women report experiencing hot flushes, they are not as common in Asian countries. It has been reported that only about 18 per cent of Chinese women[19], 15 per cent of Japanese women and 14 per cent of Singaporean women experience hot flushes.

The higher intake of dietary soy isoflavones of Japanese women compared to women in other parts of the world have been investigated as a possible explanation as to why Japanese women[20] report fewer hot flushes compared to Western women. Researchers decided to see what would happen when 100 mg of soy isoflavones was given in pill form for three months to women who were experiencing hot flushes[21]. By the end of a three-month trial the number of women experiencing hot flushes decreased from 100 per cent to only 31 per cent. The severity of their hot flushes also decreased significantly and they even reported an improvement in their mood. That sounds dramatic, and it is. The issue with this study, however, is that there was no control group (a group taking a placebo – an inactive substance) to compare with. Why is this important? Because a percentage of people are likely to experience a reduction in their hot flushes and feel better anyway due to what is called the 'placebo effect'. Even rigorously conducted hormone drug trials are required to use a control group because a large percentage of participants will also experience benefit due to the placebo effect[22].

When a well-conducted randomised control trial[23] compared the effects of soy isoflavone with those of combined oestrogen and progesterone hormone therapy and a placebo, there was no significant difference between the two types of therapies in their effectiveness of reducing hot flushes, muscle and joint aches and pains, and vaginal dryness. In other words, the soy isoflavone worked just as well as the hormone therapy.

In 2015, another large, well-regarded study[24] also looked at the effectiveness of phytoestrogens in relieving menopausal symptoms. The authors concluded that "phytoestrogens appear to reduce the frequency of hot flushes in menopausal women without serious side effects". Generally, soy products are well tolerated; however, mild symptoms of gastrointestinal bloating, nausea, diarrhoea and constipation have been reported. However, if you have an allergy to soy, **do not use any soy products.**

What about safety?

Whenever we use a medication, herbal preparation or dietary supplement, it is important that they are taken as directed. I have witnessed individuals who believe that because something is natural it is safe and that if a little (according to the directions) is helpful, then taking much larger amounts is even better. Nothing could be further from the truth. Even drinking too much water (I am talking litres of water) can be detrimental to health. Treat herbal preparations as you would any therapeutic medication: with respect, and only as directed. Using the wrong amount, using the wrong part of the herb, and/or using the herb in the wrong combination can be unsafe.

It is very important to inform your health practitioner if you are a taking herbal preparation because certain herb-drug interaction can unsafe, harmful or even toxic. Let me explain. The reason for this is that our liver changes the chemistry of drugs, converting some into more active forms and breaking others down into a more inactive forms before they are eliminated from the body. Certain herbs use the same enzyme system in the liver as several prescription drugs. The herbal compounds and the drug compounds are like a big crowd at a sports event, with supporters from two different teams all trying to push through the turnstiles (the enzyme pathway) at the same time and this causes problems. For example, St John's wort, a herbal medicine with antidepressant effects when used on its own has an encouraging safety profile however, when used at the same time as other drugs that use the same liver enzyme pathways, dangerous interactions have been reported. The bottom line is, always let your health professional know if you are using CAM therapies.

What women want

So why might women who experience distressing symptoms during their transitioning years persist with CAM therapies, particularly herbal products and plant-based compounds, despite a dearth of research into their effectiveness and questions about their safety? When perimenopausal women have been invited to share their opinions[25], the results have been enlightening and many a medical professional would do well to become acquainted with the reasons as to why a perimenopausal woman might consider using a complementary and alternative (CAM) therapy before considering an allopathic (medical) treatment. Many participants explained they considered menopause as a naturally occurring stage in life rather than a medical condition, and their choice to use CAM is regarded as health promoting in terms of both menopause and normal aging. There were concerns about prescribed medication side effects and risks associated with HRT. A sense of personal control regarding decision making as to whether or not to use medical or CAM therapies or the option to use both was highly regarded. In fact, a number of those interviewed with a preference for CAM therapies would not rule out seeing a medical doctor altogether; their preference was to first manage their symptoms using self-prescribed herbs, then approach a CAM practitioner for assistance, and if the CAM therapy was ineffective or the CAM practitioner's advice was not helpful, then a consultation with their doctor was the next step.

In my experience, women in perimenopause really want to be heard; they want to have the opportunity to discuss their options and preferences and voice their concerns with their doctor without feeling ignored, dismissed or denigrated. I invite you to make that appointment and have that discussion with your trusted health professional.

Jo, I hope you find this helpful.

Best wishes for your good health,

Dr Rosie

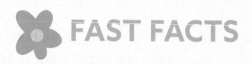
FAST FACTS

Bioidentical hormones

Bioidentical hormones are defined by the Endocrine Society as "compounds that have exactly the same chemical and molecular structure as hormones that are produced in the human body"[26]. Compound bioidentical hormones are often thought of as natural as they are based on plants such as soy or wild yam, but they are still synthesised in a laboratory – and 'natural' doesn't necessarily mean 'safe'.

There is an assumption that bioidentical hormones deliver the same benefits as HRT without any of the potential risks, but as bioidentical hormones are not approved by the Australian Therapeutics Goods Administration (TGA), there is no regulation of production quality, purity, concentration, and dosage of the contents. A review of the efficacy of bioidentical hormones concluded that "No data are yet available about the safety of bioidentical hormone therapy with regard to long-term outcomes such as heart attack, stroke and breast cancer."[27] It would seem logical that the same risks attributed to HRT be attributed to bioidentical hormones also. At this stage, there have been no studies which demonstrate otherwise.

Non-hormonal medications

Several pharmaceutical medications have been shown to help with reducing the distress of hot flushes and night sweats. These include escitalopram, citalopram, and venlafaxine, all commonly prescribed antidepressants; clonidine, a medication used to lower blood pressure; and gabapentin, which is an anticonvulsant. These medications are being used 'off-label' when used to manage symptoms of menopause; meaning they are being used outside the original purpose for which they were approved by the TGA. As for any medication, you will need to speak with your doctor as to whether this type of therapy is suitable for you in your situation and consider any negative side effects.

Complementary and Alternative Medicine (CAM) therapies

CAM therapies are those which are not typically part of conventional, Westernised health care practices. Complementary therapies are used together with conventional medicine; alternative therapies are used instead of conventional medicine. CAM therapies can be grouped under three broad categories:

- natural products (herbs, vitamins, minerals, dietary supplements)
- mind-body practices (hypnosis, meditation, CBT)
- whole-system approaches (acupuncture, traditional Chinese medicine, homeopathy).

While many women who use CAM believe them to be very helpful, results from controlled trials and large scientific reviews have been mixed. Mind-body practices were found to be safe and largely effective in managing and reducing stress and some physical symptoms; studies into the effectiveness of natural products were less conclusive. Always advise your health practitioner if you are using or thinking of using CAM therapies.

Some helpful websites and resources:

National Centre for Complementary and Integrative Health
Herbs at a Glance: https://www.nccih.nih.gov/health/herbsataglance

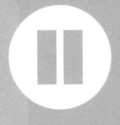

Chapter 9
INSOMNIA

Counting sheep

My first recollection of sleep deprivation was as a young child, the night before I returned to a new school year. Daylight savings played havoc with my need to sleep before the sun set. The excitement of a new teacher, classroom, friends, uniform, school bag, pencils and books meant my siblings and I were wired and unable to sleep. We would eventually give in to resistance and pass out from counting sheep once the sun was down.

My next experience was in my tweens. I spent many nights dreaming about whom I could love or who didn't love me. My young broken heart felt like it would never heal and my mum found pleasure in reminding me 'there's plenty of fish in the sea'. I would lie awake for hours, twiddling my thumbs and staring at the shadows on the ceiling whilst tossing and turning, and counting sheep into their *thousands*.

As a teenager, sleep was the least of my priorities. There was plenty of time to 'sleep when you're dead', as I thought, plus the fear of missing out on something was greater than the need to sleep. I became nocturnal and chose to follow my mum's sleeping habits. By the afternoons I'd struggle to keep my eyes open, which translated into a lack of learning and I spent my high-school days yawning and dragging my feet. It was typical for me to feel sleep-deprived and generally exhausted.

When I fell pregnant in Year 11, I managed to slip under the radar for 25 weeks! I most certainly didn't associate my extra tiredness with pregnancy, and neither did anyone else in my family.

When my babies came along, I was exhausted for at least a decade. I'm sure I can speak for all mums by saying sleep deprivation becomes part of your daily routine. I learnt to accept limited sleep and was content to achieve four hours of uninterrupted sleep a night. By the time my head hit the pillow I was out like a light – no counting sheep required during that phase. As my babies grew, I would lie awake questioning my parenting skills and amaze myself at how productive I could be with such little sleep per night, per week, per month, per year!

Having teenagers and young adults meant sleeping with one eye open until they were home safe and sound in bed. There was always a party in the middle of Woop Woop that called for an unplanned late-night pickup. Having kids with P-plate licences added to the restless and stressful evenings worrying about the potential of car accidents, drink driving, drug use and even suicide.

Since the kids have flown the coop, I've maintained a regular sleeping pattern and I'm proud to say I'm no longer nocturnal. I'm down with the sun and up with the chooks, and bounce out of bed feeling fantastic to start a new day. I seek pleasure from watching the sunrise and eventually got over the need to stay up late for no particular reason.

So now, I have the luxury to sleep and nap whenever I like; no babies to keep me up, no teenagers to pick up, no broken heart to heal, but those bloody sheep have recently re-entered my nocturnal bliss and there are just so many of them!

I try to maintain a relaxing routine before bed; and I *fall* asleep easily. But I'm woken in the early hours, saturated in sweat from head to toe, and needing to wee. My legs are restless, and I practise controlled-breathing techniques and meditation as I lie awake contemplating my next move. Should I give in and get up, turn on the light and read a book, watch a movie or check my news feed, take another herbal compound ... but it's madness at 2 a.m. My girlfriend refers to this time as the 'witching hours', which translates into becoming a witch if this lifestyle continues. I've heard about the 3 a.m. club – that's full of middle-aged women prowling the online forums and playing Candy Crush until nearly dawn!

Finally, after a couple of hours of over-analysing everything in my life and trying to solve all the problems of the world, I drift off to sleep only to be woken by an irritating alarm. I drag myself out of bed after pressing the snooze button three times, exhausted from another night of broken sleep and the thought of what lies ahead. My zest for life has diminished, and I'm not interested in watching the sunrise today, although there are places to go and people to see. I live in hope that tonight I will fall into a deep sleep and wake uninterrupted seven hours later.

It's a cruel irony and I try to rationalise what keeps me awake. I have nothing to worry about but I'm back to where I started as a new mum, experiencing broken sleep night after night. Without a decent night's sleep, I'm snappy, irritable and losing control. My natural glow is long gone, and you could pack a week's worth of baggage into the bags under my eyes. Fatigue is now affecting all aspects of my life and I crave sugar and caffeine to give myself the boost I need to make it through the days. It affects my relationships, kidnaps my patience and tolerance – no wonder I'm snappy. Sleep deprivation is cumulative and debilitating; it steals what remains of your memory after dropping oestrogen levels have already raided the supply.

My body is adrift at sea, unravelling on its own accord. I encounter fleeting moments of my former self that are melting before me and I wonder when it will end. So, if 'for every physical there's an emotional'.

Maybe what I need to do is lose control completely; let go, cherish the here and now rather than focusing on what was. Easier said than done!

Rather than counting sheep, I've decided to embrace my new mantra: 'let go, let go, let go, let go, let go' and pray that soon I will fall back into a blissful slumber and wake bright, refreshed and keen to watch the sunrise again.

Dear Dr Rosie

- Why do perimenopausal women experience insomnia?
- What can I do to support my own sleep patterns?
- What if I need extra help, are there therapies or medications I can try?

Honestly, as if we haven't sacrificed enough of ourselves over the years!

Thanks, Jo

Let's talk about insomnia

Dear Jo,

If there is one thing that will turn a mild-mannered woman into a self-confessed witch, it is most likely to be the wide-eyed wakefulness of insomnia. Whether it is difficulty getting to sleep, problems with staying asleep or early-morning waking, it seems that disrupted sleep is a common problem during perimenopause[1].

Restorative sleep is like a reboot for our brain, restoring our brain energy, consolidating our learning by moving short term memory into long-term storage, and taking out the trash of brain waste products[2] that build up during the day. Not getting sufficient zzzz's can reduce our quality of life, interfere with our daytime functioning and affect our mental and physical health now and in the future. We might wake with a groggy head and need that heart-starter coffee to get things going in the morning, but many people find they don't deal with minor irritations as easily as their well-slept colleagues. Mood can be affected with the apparent two-way relationship between insomnia and depressed mood[3]. The enjoyment factor in our social engagements with family members and friends may decrease. We may find that it takes more effort to concentrate and complete work tasks and we end up making more errors.

Why do perimenopausal women experience insomnia?

Is insomnia in women at this time of life prevalent because they are often bothered by hot flushes, night sweats and clammy chills? The bottom line is that sleep difficulties appear to increase with age[4]. The US SWAN study[5] looked at sleep during perimenopause and found that perimenopausal women experience disturbed sleep even without the distress of hot flushes. During perimenopause an estimated 32 to 47 per cent of women report that they have problems with sleep compared with women before they hit perimenopause (16 to 42 per cent). For those who have entered either a natural or surgical menopause, the number rises to between 35 and 60 per cent. However, the good news is that, therefore, more than 40 per cent of women going through either the transition or menopause itself have no issues with poor sleep.

Restorative REM sleep

Sleep is made up four stages, three stages of non-rapid eye movement (NREM), which is the deep restorative phase, and rapid eye movement (REM) sleep. Over the course of the night you normally progress through a these four stages between four and six times. As we age, we tend to spend less time in deep NREM sleep. Sleep studies show that being woken by hot flushes is more common during the first four hours of getting to sleep during NREM sleep and that REM sleep in the second half of the night supresses hot flushes and the associated wakening[6]. As we normally tend to spend only 20 to 25 percent of total sleep time in REM[7], it can be frustrating to be woken by a hot flush, a bladder that needs to be emptied or the joint aches and muscle pains associated with changing oestrogen levels.

Hormones

Sleep researchers suggest that it is not simply declining levels of oestrogen but the *rate* of change in those hormones that influence sleep. The Melbourne Women's Midlife Health Project[8] discovered that a sharper decline in oestrogen levels was associated with greater severity of sleep problems. At the same time, there are other age-related decreases in growth hormone, prolactin and melatonin which may also be contributing to perimenopausal sleep disturbance[9]. Progesterone also declines. Progesterone has a sleep-inducing effect, increasing the production of GABA, a brain neurotransmitter that helps the mind to relax, fall asleep and sleep soundly[10]. Melatonin is released by the pineal gland in our brain and this light-sensitive body clock regulates our sleep–wake circadian cycle. Our natural circadian sleep–wake cycle is just over 24 hours long. Shift work, jet lag, late night blue light emissions from our mobile phone, e-book or computer screens switches off melatonin, which then disrupts our normal circadian rhythm.

Although hot flushes often get the blame for disturbed sleep, there may be other biological, endocrine, psychological, social or behavioural factors that are contributing to the issue and need addressing.

Other reasons for insomnia

Medical conditions include movement disorders when your legs won't keep still; breathing disorders such as obstructive sleep apnoea (definitely get this checked out if your partner tells you that you snore or you have stopped breathing during the night, or you wake yourself gasping for air); the rising discomfort of gastric reflux; the dull, foggy head of sinus infection or allergies; and joint or muscle aches such as the pains associated with arthritis, low back pain and fibromyalgia. These can all interfere with sleep and also contribute to depression.

Medications for some conditions such as antihypertensives for high blood pressure, antihistamines for sinus issues, and thyroid medications, can also interfere with sleep. It may be helpful to make an appointment with your doctor to check if there are any underlying treatable medical issues and whether any medications you are currently taking may be contributing to your sleepless nights.

Overdoing alcohol can have you waking in the middle of the night. Initially, intoxication can see us crashing into bed, but as the level of alcohol in our blood decreases over the next few hours, we often wake in the early hours of the morning. Not only can alcohol disrupt our natural circadian sleep–wake cycle and block restorative REM sleep, but its diuretic effect can mean you need to get up to empty your bladder. It has been said that more people are woken by a full bladder than by their alarm clock.

Taking our troubles to bed can have us lying awake clock-watching: 1 a.m., 2 a.m. ... 5 a.m. Have you ever tumbled into bed at the end of the day, exhausted and struggling to keep your eyes open, and then those worrying thoughts start circling? Concerns about getting that report written, your ageing parent's latest health crisis, a Year 12 adolescent preparing for exams, financial worries, relationship issues ... round and round like a sushi train it goes. The things you wish you had said, the things you wish you could un-say, scripting and re-scripting those must-have-one-day conversations, going over and over those step-by-step plans for tomorrow.

Insomnia can also be a conditioned response. It can happen that going to bed and turning off the lights can become an automatic trigger to insomnia. Perhaps initially, you were woken by the discomfort of hot flushes and night sweats, and so by now you have associated this with not being able to get a good night's sleep. Or perhaps switching off the light triggers those concerns you feel quite capable of dealing with during daylight hours but now they appear almost insurmountable in the dark, devoid of distraction.

The good news is that insomnia is treatable and there are a range of options available, from the do-it-yourself variety to cognitive behavioural training and prescription medications. I have already mentioned a few tips you may like to try. Remember, there is no one-size-fits-all remedy and sometimes it's a matter of trying out what best suits you.

What we know is that generally people prefer non-pharmacological methods to improve their sleep and medical guidelines recommend the use of cognitive and behavioural therapies, which have been shown to be effective, with medication as a last resort.

It is important to ensure you are getting sufficient shut-eye because insufficient or poor-quality sleep is associated with a greater likelihood of developing physical and mental health issues such as obesity, depression, heart disease and diabetes[11,12,13].

How to support your sleep patterns

Establishing helpful sleep routines and healthy lifestyle habits can support a regular sleep pattern.

Develop some helpful routines for sleep

- Go to bed at the same time each night and only sleep long enough to feel rested.
- Get up at the same time every day.
- Ride the sleep wave. Sleep comes in cycles, so if you are unable to get to sleep within 15 to 30 minutes, don't stay in bed. Get up out of bed and try again later.
- Remove all electronic devices from the bedroom.
- Monitor your consumption of caffeine, food, alcohol and cigarettes.

Consider your caffeine intake because it may be keeping you awake at night. Coffee has psychoactive properties to keep our mind alert. It reaches its peak effect about one hour after we drink it and keeps us going for around four to six hours before the effect wears off. In some people the caffeine may take up to 24 hours to be eliminated from their bodies. How much caffeine is in a cup of coffee depends on the brand and the strength: one shot or two? As a guide, a 250 mL cup of instant coffee contains about 100 mg of caffeine, whereas brewed barista coffee may contain anywhere from 50 to 350 mg per cup. And don't forget those caffeinated sugary drinks because they can have the same effect. It's best to avoid caffeine if insomnia is an issue. However, if you are unable to give up coffee, then consider reducing your intake to no more than two cups a day (around 200 mg of caffeine); do not have caffeine for at least four hours before going to bed and preferably not after midday.

Whilst we are talking about what we put in our mouth, consider not eating a large or spicy meal at least three hours before trying to go to sleep. It takes time for our body to digest food so make your evening meal light and preferably finished by 6 p.m.

Alcohol can initially be relaxing; however, the sudden drop in blood sugar levels may prompt your body to wake. And although many people like to smoke before they head to bed, in fact the nicotine has a stimulating effect.

Teas and tisanes

If you do want non-caffeinated, non-alcoholic drink before bed, consider a herbal tea. The use of herbal teas to combat insomnia is common, despite some of those teas said to have a taste of straw or old socks. Effectiveness and safety of any remedy, whether natural or synthesised, are always issues to consider. Whilst many people swear by their nightly soothing cup of herbal tea, clinical trials[14] which have subjected herbs to scientific evaluation, have, on the whole, not demonstrated that they are more effective than placebo, and more research is required.

The challenge with research into herbal remedies is that clinical studies rely on standardising the herb which means that every batch must be identical. Widespread standardisation is never going to be possible 'in the real world' because a herb's composition may vary from batch to batch due to differences in the part of the plant used to be tested (flowers, seeds, stem, bark, roots), the time of harvesting, the country of origin and how long it has been stored. Further, whilst an active ingredient of a herb may be patented (and make money for the patent-holder), a whole herb is unable to be patented. As research trials are expensive to set up and run, there is not much incentive to study a therapy that cannot be patented or provide a substantial return on investment. Reassuringly, studies have provided evidence demonstrating the safety of valerian, hops, German chamomile and passionflower so you may happily sip away on your soothing night-time cuppa[15].

There are numerous herbs that have historically been used to promote a calming effect and induce sleep but some of the more popular ones include:

- **Valerian** *(Valeriana officinalis)*
- **Chamomile** *(Matricaria chamomilla)*
- **Hops** *(Humulus lupulus)*
- **Passionflower** *(Passiflora incarnata)*
- **Skullcap** *(Scutellaria lariflora)*
- **Lemon balm** *(Melissa officinalis)*
- **Peppermint** *(Mentha x piperita)*

Actually, the word *tea* refers to the black or green tea varieties that come from a specific evergreen shrub, *Camellia sinensis*. If we are to be more correct, a *tisane* is an infusion made by steeping the softer parts of the herb, which includes the leaves, flowers, soft seeds or stem, whilst a *decoction* is made by boiling the woodier roots and/or bark.

The method for preparing a herbal tisane is to use two teaspoons of loose herb for every person, add hot water and allow the herb to steep for three to five minutes. It is best drunk 30 to 60 minutes before heading to bed.

With more research required into their effectiveness, you might wonder how you can determine if a herbal tisane is right for you. Think about what a good night's sleep means for you. For some people, getting a good night's sleep means seven to eight hours of uninterrupted shuteye; some who wake at 2 a.m. or 3 a.m. consider getting back to sleep quickly to be their goal, whilst for others a having a good night's sleep simply means waking refreshed no matter the circumstances. This underlines the fact that we are all different.

Next, rate what your 'good night' target value is for you. Does that mean you achieve your particular sleep goal 50 per cent of the time, 60 per cent or 80 per cent over the next 10 days?

Trial your nightly soothing cuppa and track your sleep over 10 days.

Review how you went. At the end of your 'trial of therapy', see if you have achieved your goal: Yes? No? Maybe? If at the end you remain unsure, you may like to continue for a little while longer, or perhaps try something different.

Create a sleep-promoting environment

Create a restful sleep environment that does not overstimulate your senses and make a commitment to yourself to keep the bedroom for sleep and sex, not watching television or typing on your laptop.

Light

Dim your lights at least two hours before bedtime, and it is recommended you avoid looking at screens such as mobile phones, e-books and computers. Our internal body clock runs on a sleep–wake cycle, which is about 24 hours long and responds to light in the environment. The sleep–wake cycle also influences our eating habits, digestion and hormone release[16]. Apparently, two hours of exposure to blue light at night will delay the release of the hormone melatonin, which helps us to feel sleepy, and will therefore disrupt our circadian rhythm. Although fluorescent and LED lights are more energy efficient, they also produce more blue light. And consider keeping night lights to a minimum or wearing an eye pillow as even exposure to low-level light (5–10 lx) with eyes closed elicits a circadian response[17].

Sometimes it can be as simple as not charging your phone or tablet in the bedroom.

KATE

Kate (51) is a coffee barista who was having difficulty getting to sleep and then staying asleep due to the light on her mobile phone and middle-of-the-night updates.

"Disturbed sleep was a problem for me. I committed to leaving my mobile charging in the kitchen and converting to an old-fashioned alarm clock in the bedroom. I used a chart on my fridge to map my progress. It was challenging at first because I had not realised that I had been in the habit of playing Candy Crush before turning out the light. When I started to see all the ticked boxes on my chart on my fridge door, I was pretty pleased with myself. But when I started sleeping through the night and waking up feeling more refreshed, I was amazed that something as simple as leaving my mobile out of the bedroom could have made such a difference to my health. Sometimes, I wonder why I had not thought of doing it sooner."

Light therapy

When the normal circadian sleep-wake cycle is out of whack, timed exposure to bright light has been used successfully to manage shift work, jet lag, delayed sleep onset issue and irregular sleep-wake rhythm[18].

Sound

Some people can sleep like a rock whilst others are highly sensitive to sound and disrupted by a pin dropping. Sounds as low as 30 decibels can affect sleep. Apparently, the most likely time when sleep is disrupted is during the light stage two of non-REM sleep. You may like to consider earplugs or a white noise generator to cancel out environmental noise and improve your sleep quality.

Touch and temperature

Choose a comfortable mattress and pillow to cuddle up with. Naturally breathable cotton sheets and PJs help decrease sweaty discomfort. Open windows and keep air circulating with fans, either portable or ceiling-mounted.

What if you're still having problems?

If do-it-yourself lifestyle changes and regular sleep routines are not enough, then consider a visit to your GP for a sleep assessment and a supervised action plan for sleep restriction therapy, relaxation therapy, mindfulness meditation and/or CBT-I.

Sleep restriction therapy

The purpose of this therapy is to improve your length and quality of sleep. It means that you will spend less time in bed worrying and wakeful. However, it does take some dedication and work on your part because you are training your body to a new way of associating bed with restful restorative sleep.

Relaxation therapies

Techniques such as deep breathing, progressive muscle relaxation, visualisation and imagery are used to deal with physical tension, help to derail the sushi train of worrying thoughts and a racing mind.

Mindfulness meditation

This is another effective drug-free solution to put the brakes on the sushi train of circling thoughts in our head as we worry about the past or stress about the future. Mindfulness helps us to remain in the present and observe our thoughts in a non-judgemental way.

Referral to a psychologist can be arranged to assist with these techniques in addition to cognitive behavioural therapy specifically structured and approved for treating insomnia called CBT-I with the 'I' designation for insomnia. CBT-I is available as a stand-alone therapy or in combination with medication.

Cognitive behavioural therapy for insomnia (CBT-I)

CBT-I uses a combination of sleep hygiene practices to help create an environment that will promote sleep, including sleep restriction, and helps to adjust our dysfunctional beliefs associated with our bed and sleep. You may be surprised to discover you are already using some of these strategies.

CBT-I targets the thoughts and behaviours that contribute to insomnia and is an effective drug-free treatment; in some cases this is more effective than medication in the short term and has benefits in the longer term[19]. A randomised control trial involving 106 perimenopausal and menopausal women who experienced two or more hot flushes daily and suffered with insomnia were divided into two groups[20]. The group receiving CBT-I by telephone for eight weeks reported a greater improvement in sleep quality than the group who did not have this intervention. Interestingly, there was no decrease in the frequency and severity of hot flushes or how troubling the hot flushes were for the CBT-I group, but they were able to function better during the day and most likely get to sleep more easily after waking during the night. The downside is that CBT-I can be time-consuming (four to eight weeks) and it does require you to do your homework. There are a couple of ways to access this help. One is to get a referral from your doctor to a psychologist who promotes CBT-I as a treatment. When I attempted to organise this referral for a face-to-face consultation for a patient, the nearest clinic was over 500 kilometres away. This lack of access is an issue for people living in regional or remote locations and as many people are time-poor, lack of convenience is another issue. There are several online options such as Slumber Pro, Sleepio, SHUTi and CBT-I Coach available which tick the boxes for access and time management, but is an online platform as effective as face-to-face sessions? A large meta-analysis review[21] found that this method of online access can provide meaningful improvements of sleep issues and is comparable to in-person sessions.

Melatonin

Melatonin is a natural hormone released by our brain's pineal gland in response to light and darkness that controls our natural sleep–wake cycle. We release melatonin at night to help us get to sleep and stay asleep. The production of melatonin by the pineal gland declines with age with a sharp drop during perimenopause before menopause occurs[22].

Light in the morning inactivates melatonin so that we wake. However, artificial disruptions may interfere with our normal circadian cycle as we travel across time zones, do shift-work or are exposed late at night to blue light emitted from mobile phones, computers, eBooks and tablets. Melatonin declines naturally during the perimenopausal transition[23].

Melatonin is available in either a 6x homeopathic supplement form from health food shops and chemists, or as a longer acting pharmaceutical medication on prescription from the doctor, marketed as a 2mg slow-release tablet in Australia.

Although a melatonin supplement may be used in the short term to improve both sleep quality and mental alertness the next day, it is more useful for resetting the body clock disrupted by jet lag rather than as a treatment for chronic insomnia. Timing the administration of crushed prolonged release melatonin together with light therapy (mentioned above) has been successfully used to reset disrupted sleep-wake cycle[24].

As with any medications, some people do experience side effects and sometimes (less than 1 in 100 people) report an increase in their insomnia, anxiety and abnormal dreams. Remember, everyone is different and what works for one person may not be suitable for another.

Pharmacological medications

Lastly, a word of caution about the use of sleep medications which include benzodiazepines, and non-benzodiazepines such as sedating antidepressants, antipsychotics and antihistamines. Although people may resort to such medications to break their pattern of insomnia, or for a quick fix when they are truly desperate, this should only ever be a short-term solution because in the long term, sleeping pills can do more harm than good. Concerns with benzodiazepines include addiction and tolerance (needing to take more of the medication to produce the same effect). Non-benzo sleep medications include antidepressants with sedating properties, antipsychotics and antihistamines. As with any medication, there may be side effects from these non-benzo medications which include weight gain and increased risk of developing diabetes.

Disrupted sleep is a common problem during the peri-menopause transition and a lack of refreshing sleep can interfere with our daytime functioning, really reduce our quality of life and affect our mental and physical health now and in the future. If you are having issues in this area, then please do not alone, do not suffer in silence. I encourage you to explore the options available and call on extra assistance if you need it.

Jo, I truly hope that you find this information a helpful starting point.

Yours in good health,

Dr Rosie

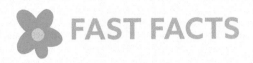 **FAST FACTS**

Insomnia and sleep deprivation

Whether it is difficulty getting to sleep, problems with staying asleep or early morning waking, it seems that disrupted sleep is a common problem during perimenopause. It has been found that 32 to 47 per cent of women who experience a natural perimenopausal transition report disturbed sleep.

Why do perimenopausal women experience insomnia?

- Hormonal changes such as declining oestrogen and progesterone levels, other age-related decreases in growth hormone, prolactin and melatonin.
- Medical conditions such as restless legs syndrome, obstructive sleep apnoea, gastric reflux.
- Some medications.
- Overdoing the alcohol, coffee, cigarettes or food.
- Taking our troubles to bed.
- A conditioned response.

Develop some helpful routines for sleep

- Go to bed at the same time each night and only sleep long enough to feel rested.
- Get up at the same time every day.
- Ride the sleep wave. Sleep comes in cycles, so if you are unable to get to sleep within 15 to 30 minutes, don't stay in bed. Get up out of bed and try again later.

- ✿ Monitor your caffeine intake and preferably do not have coffee after midday.
- ✿ Avoid smoking in the evening as nicotine has a stimulatory effect.
- ✿ Avoid alcohol where possible.
- ✿ Avoid heavy or spicy meals at least three hours before going to bed.

Teas and tisanes

The use of herbal teas such as German chamomile, valerian, hops, lemon balm, skullcap or passionflower is common when battling insomnia. They generally have no harmful side effects and they may be worth a try.

Still having problems?

Ask your GP for a sleep assessment and a supervised action plan for sleep restriction therapy, relaxation therapy, mindfulness meditation and/or CBT-I; your GP may also suggest melatonin supplements or other sleep medications.

Melatonin

Melatonin is a natural hormone released by our brain's pineal gland in response to light and darkness and controls our natural sleep–wake cycle. Melatonin declines naturally during the perimenopausal transition. Melatonin supplements may be used in the short term to improve both sleep quality and mental alertness the next day.

Pharmacological medications

A word of caution about the use of sleep medications which include benzodiazepines, and non-benzodiazepines such as sedating antidepressants, antipsychotics and antihistamines. Concerns with benzodiazepines include addiction and tolerance (needing to take more of the medication to produce the same effect). Side effects from non-benzo medications include weight gain and increased risk of developing diabetes.

Some helpful websites and resources:

Australian Sleep Health Foundation
https://www.sleephealthfoundation.org.au/

Sleep Therapy Australia
https://www.sleeptherapy.com.au/

Australian QUIT LINE 1800 QUIT or call 13 78 48
https://www.quitlinesa.org.au/

Chapter 10
VAGINAL DRYNESS

The Simpson Desert

Finding the right words to describe the change of environment in my private bits is proving challenging, and if I'm honest, denial has been an easier place to be rather than accept that my once tropical rainforest is now the Simpson Desert!

Surely a girl's an expert when it comes to the natural ebb and flow downstairs and therefore navigating our own weather pattern is normally straightforward, right?

Picture this for a moment: a lush, dense, moist, plentiful, fertile rainforest rich in biodiversity, constantly rejuvenating and recreating itself. Now, imagine this: dry, barren, dehydrated, lifeless, harsh, uninviting, dry – did I mention DRY?! OMG, my bodily fluids have dried up and my pleasure pit has become a gravel pit!

As if there aren't already enough unpleasantries associated with perimenopause, now we have yet another bodily challenge to manage.

Lovemaking shouldn't feel like carpet burn inside, although the friction caused from intercourse can make the whole 'getting down and dirty' process painful instead of pleasurable.

My girlfriend shared a funny story of experimenting with lubricants. Firstly, she believes you need a chemistry lesson to distinguish between silicon, water-based and vegan options (yes, true); some with applicators, others in squeezable tubes that have a mind of their own and leave you in a sticky fragranced mess. Her personal favourite (so she thought) was the 'his and her', until the 'fire and ice' version delivered what it promised. This adventurous activity saw 'him and her' showering to soothe and put out the fire that had erupted between their legs – oouch! And for those of us with food intolerances, I wonder if there's a gluten-free, dairy-free option available?

The moral to this story is to keep experimenting and do whatever it takes to find the lightness and fun but remember, don't believe everything you read on the packaging.

I often reflect on the life well lived and mourn the loss of the vagina that once was.

How does one begin to talk about the much loved and lived vagina?

Youthful, energetic, athletic, playful, never one to shy away from a challenge. Full of stamina and endurance with great staying power. Strong, tough, resilient to withstand the harshest conditions. Gifted to remodel and talented to spring back into shape after being bent, stretched and twisted into the most dynamic positions. Yes, flexibility and durability were her strengths – and to think I took all of this for granted!

I consider the generations of women that have gone before me with respect and reflect on my own mother, grandmothers and mother-in-law, and wonder how they coped during this time. Did they have open and honest discussions with their husbands? Did they giggle with their girlfriends? Was this 'secret women's business'? Was it easier to pretend or deny than confront? Or were they gracious in accepting 'the change' and just got on with it?

As I get used to the new norm, it's time to rewrite the narrative of my vagina by letting go of the lush rainforest and surrendering to the Simpson Desert. I have decided to take a light-hearted approach by keeping a great sense of humour, laughing lots and delving into the world of 'lubes'.

Dear Dr Rosie,

- Why has my vagina become as dry as the Simpson Desert?
- Why can lovemaking sometimes be so painful?
- Is there anything that might help?

Thanks,
Jo

Let's talk about vaginal dryness

I'm pleased that you've brought up this subject as many women suffer in silence because they feel excruciatingly uncomfortable discussing this 'downstairs' area of sexual health with their doctor. In fact, lots of women don't talk about their concerns with *anyone* – not their intimate partner, not their friends ... no-one.

Why has my vagina become so dry?

There are a couple of reasons midlife women experience vaginal dryness. One is to do with biological changes that start to occur during perimenopause and the second reason is to do with issues involving sexual arousal.

Oestrogen and lubrication

As oestrogen levels are more erratic during the perimenopause and tend not to stay at a stable low level until after the final menstrual period, most women during the transition phase are usually unaffected. In a study[1] of Australian perimenopausal women, 4 per cent reported that they had an issue with vaginal dryness. In the year after the final menstrual period this will jump up to 25 per cent and three years later, well and truly into menopause, the figure is 47 per cent. In the long term, more than 50 per cent of menopausal women experience this issue.

From a purely biological view, our body is changing hormonally and physically. During our younger years, under the influence of oestrogen, the cells lining the vagina are plumped up with glycogen (a compound made in the body to store glucose). Now, we all know how much we love sugar and the good *Lactobacillus* bacteria that reside in our vagina are no different. These glycogen-rich lining cells are shed into the vagina and release glucose, which feeds the healthy *Lactobacillus* species populations. The good bacteria produce a moderately acidic mucus, a natural lubricant that keeps unhealthy bacteria and *Candida* yeasts (which can cause thrush) under control. There really is a lush tropical ecosystem down there!

Sometimes women are concerned about having a vaginal discharge. It is perfectly normal to have a small amount of white discharge that ranges from thinner and wetter to thicker and tackier over the course of the menstrual cycle – you've no doubt noticed it at times during your adult life. However, if you develop a vaginal discharge that has an unusual grey, white or green look to it, smells 'a bit fishy' or foul, or your vagina burns when you pee or gets itchy, you should have this checked out by your doctor.

Changes start to occur around our mid to late forties as oestrogen declines and the glycogen in vaginal lining cells also decreases. The vaginal lining cells that were previously pumped up with glycogen now become thinner; and with less natural lubrication, we may start to experience vaginal dryness, irritation, burning or itching, and even the occasional vaginal thrush outbreak.

Lubrication relies on hormones and a healthy blood supply. Oestrogen also helps maintain the elasticity of the vaginal tissues. Bartholin's glands, located near the vagina entrance, also deliver extra fluid into the vagina for lubrication when a woman is aroused. When oestrogen declines, collagen in the vaginal walls decreases and hence there is a loss of elasticity; and the Bartholin's glands don't lubricate as much. And then there is a decrease in the blood flow to the vulvo-vaginal area which previously helped the vagina and clitoris get all hot and bothered and ready for action.

Sexual arousal

With sexual arousal, there is increased blood flow to the vaginal tissues, and vaginal intercourse gives vaginal muscles a workout to maintain vaginal width, length and tone, and stimulates lubricating fluids to keep it moist downstairs. But don't forget the clitoris (which has the same evolutionary origin as the penis), rich in blood supply and nerve endings, is the main player when it comes to orgasm. When oestrogen levels decrease there is reduction in the blood flow and clitoris nerve sensation, which means less sensitivity and less lubrication[2]. In the early stages of perimenopause, one of the first signs of lowered oestrogen levels may simply be a slight decrease in lubrication on sexual arousal. Although everything may still be in working order, it can often be a matter of taking a bit of extra time in the lead up to the main event to get the juices flowing.

Remember, during perimenopause there are still ups and downs in the level of ovarian oestrogen, so the juices downstairs tend to fluctuate before the oestrogen levels take a dive downwards. For many women transitioning to menopause, the vaginal dryness associated with intercourse is due to insufficient arousal.

So, relax. Take a breath. Take your time. Explore. This does not have to be a race to the finish line. In the next chapter, we'll talk a bit more about your libido and how that might be involved too.

Why can lovemaking sometimes be so painful during perimenopause?

Dyspareunia is medical-speak for discomfort or pain associated with intercourse, and for about 18 per cent[3] to 20 per cent[4] of perimenopausal women this is sometimes an issue, with vaginal dryness highly associated with pain. The combination of the lack of effective lubrication together with a fraction too much friction during intercourse can result in this discomfort or pain.

Women who experience vaginal dryness are more likely to experience dyspareunia, have difficulties with sexual arousal and culmination in orgasm, and feel less emotional sexual satisfaction. However, it has been noted that in spite of these issues, the frequency of sexual activity tends not to change[5]. And the good news is that regular vaginal sexual activity, either with your partner or going solo, can help with vaginal dryness.

Is there anything that might help?

You may find that you need that extra bit of help by using a vaginal lubricant and/or vaginal moisturiser. That's right; moisturisers are not only for our face. Stay with me, Jo, and we will explore this further.

Vaginal lubricants

Lubricants simply lubricate; they do not plump up the vaginal lining, but they do help everything slip and slide more easily. These over-the-counter products come in a variety of options from water-based lubricants to plant-based oils such as olive oil or sweet almond oil, to other commercially produced mineral oil-based products. The old Vaseline was perhaps the mainstay of our grandparents' era, and more recently, almond or coconut oil is being promoted by those wanting natural options. It is mostly a matter of personal choice and trial to find what suits. Water-based options are the go if you are using a condom as oil-based lubricants will cause condom materials to perish.

Lubricants are applied just before intercourse in and around the vaginal area to the vulva, the part that touches your under-wear, and includes the outer part of the vagina including the two sets of lips at the entrance and the clitoris. Additionally, drawing up the lubricant into a small syringe and using it as a 'lubricant launcher' to insert the product inside the vagina may be helpful. Some people apply this to their partner's penis as part of foreplay because it feels less clinical to them, whereas others prefer to get ready on their own. It's up to you.

Vaginal moisturisers

Vaginal moisturisers are non-hormonal vaginal creams that have been reported to reduce symptoms of dryness, itching, burning and discomfort. They are a different thing from lubricants, and they have the ability to retain water, which is then gradually released in the vagina to mimic the normal vaginal secretions. Moisturisers are not applied 'at the scene of the action' but instead they are applied two to three times a week and last for about two days. This can be helpful for women who are not sexually active and suffering with vaginal discomfort.

Low-dose vaginal oestrogen

Vaginal oestrogen in the form of a cream or pessary (a tablet inserted into the vagina) is a form of very low dose hormone replacement therapy (HRT) which acts locally on vaginal tissues. Vaginal low dose HRT is body identical, which means that oestrogen used is in the form of oestradiol, which is the same as the oestrogen made in our ovaries and therefore classed as a natural oestrogen.

The benefits of using this form of oestrogen is that researchers have found there is very low absorption into the bloodstream and therefore the addition of progesterone to ensure uterine health is not required. A review of 53 different clinical trials[6] found low dose vaginal oestrogen to be effective in relieving vaginal dryness and generally safe with few side effects. The main side effects to watch for are breast tenderness and vaginal bleeding. Be aware that if, at any time, you experience abnormal vaginal bleeding, you must be reviewed by your doctor.

Lifestyle strategies

There are also some simple lifestyle strategies you can consider if you're experiencing vaginal dryness and discomfort.

You may find you feel more comfortable wearing underwear made of natural fibres like cotton or bamboo, rather than synthetic fabrics, which hold the moisture close to your skin and thereby set up an environment where yeast infections are more likely to grow.

Consider avoiding perfumed vaginal hygiene products that potentially irritate sensitive vaginal tissues and upset the pH balance that keeps yeast and bacterial infections under control. Some women find that using a perfumed deodorant or vaginal hygiene spray or soap doesn't cause them any problem, but if you do tend to get dry or irritated downstairs, using water or a mild unscented soap to wash the area around the vagina (the vulva) is fine to keep your lady bits clean. Talcum powder, bubble bath, perfumed toilet tissues and panty liners are best avoided also.

Some women use a douche, which is the process of cleansing the inside of the vagina for aesthetic reasons, cultural reasons, or with the intention of preventing or treating an infection and cleansing after menstruating. However, douching is associated with several negative effects, including upsetting the normally low pH (4.5) balance of a woman's vaginal tissues and predisposing her to vaginal infection such as bacterial vaginosis, vaginal candidiasis, pelvic inflammatory disease and ectopic pregnancy. The bottom line is, women are advised not to douche. However, given the entrenchment of cultural and behavioural norms in some areas of the world, many women will choose to continue this practice.

Research[7] also indicates that diet may play a role, with phytoestrogens associated with a modest improvement vaginal dryness. Soy is a great source of phytoestrogens, and a diet rich in soy foods would include tofu, soy milk and edamame (whole soybeans). Including plenty of fresh or lightly cooked and fermented veggies, yoghurt and other

Lactobacillus foods in your diet will also help to ensure your vaginal rainforest remains resilient.

The vaginal microbiome

Now, we have spoken about declining oestrogen levels, but the vaginal microbiome is an area that is generating a lot of interest in the scientific community. You spoke of a lush rainforest ecology in the vagina, and Jo, you are correct. We know that bacteria were first discovered by Dutch scientist Antonie van Leeuwenhoek as he peered through his microscope in the 1670s. In 2012, the Human Microbiome Project mapped the microbial makeup of different body sites such as the skin, mouth, nose, lower gut and vagina.

Researchers found that different areas of the body host different taxonomic groups and numbers of bacteria. *Lactobacillus* bacteria are an important colonising type of bacteria found in a healthy vagina that ferment the glycogen made in vaginal lining cells, producing lactic acid to help keep the environment at an acidic pH of less than 4.5. This acidity helps prevent the unfavourable overgrowth growth of yeasts such as *Candida albicans* and *Candida glabrata* and keep bacterial infections such as bacterial vaginosis which is the one that causes a discharge with a fishy smell, under control.

Microbial diversity

The numerous types of microbial populations have been likened to a rainforest ecosystem and highlighted the importance of many species coexisting in mutually beneficial ways to maintain the health of the rainforest.

Studies show that microbial diversity is important for maintaining a healthy gut ecosystem and, as it happens, also for maintaining a healthy vaginal ecosystem. Diversity is made up of:

- richness (the number of different microbial species)
- evenness (the relative proportion of each microbe species)

The reason diversity is important is to allow your body to bounce back quickly from a disturbance such as an infection by harmful bacteria (as opposed to the good bacteria) that requires a course of antibiotics to control. Antibiotics can be lifesaving and necessary to treat serious infections such as a bacterial chest infection, but they are not appropriate for a viral infection. Some antibiotics have a very narrow-targeted action – like a chemical laser beam – and only kill off those particular germs, while other antibiotics have a much broader spectrum of action; they work a bit like a scatter gun so they end up not only wiping out the bad bacteria that are causing your chest infection but also may wipe out some of your good gut and vaginal bacteria. An oral probiotic taken at least two or three hours away from an antibiotic dose and continued for two to four weeks afterwards helps maintain healthy vaginal flora and decrease the likelihood of a vaginal yeast infection.

✳

Jo, I hope you find this helpful.

Best wishes for your good health,

Dr Rosie

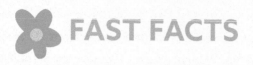 **FAST FACTS**

Why has my vagina become so dry?

Vaginal dryness may be due to the biological changes that start to occur during menopause, and issues involving sexual arousal. When oestrogen declines, collagen in the vaginal walls decreases and there is a loss of elasticity and the Bartholin's glands don't lubricate as much. There is also a decrease in the blood flow to the vulvo-vaginal area which previously helped the vagina and clitoris get ready for action. In the early stages of perimenopause, one of the first signs of lowering oestrogen levels may simply be a slight decrease in lubrication on sexual arousal. Relax. Take your time.

An Australian study found around 4 per cent of perimenopausal women report vaginal dryness as an issue, with the percentage had increasing to 25 per cent one year after the final menstrual period. In the long term, more than 50 per cent of menopausal women experience this issue.

Why is lovemaking sometimes so painful?

The combination of lack of effective lubrication together with a fraction too much friction can result in discomfort or pain associated with intercourse, which is known as *dyspareunia*.

Women who experience vaginal dryness are more likely to experience dyspareunia, have difficulties with sexual arousal and culmination in orgasm, and feel less emotional sexual satisfaction.

What are the options to manage this issue?

- Vaginal lubricants
- Vaginal moisturisers
- Low-dose oestrogen vaginal cream or pessary
- Lifestyle strategies

Lifestyle strategies include wearing underwear made of natural fibres like cotton or bamboo, rather than synthetics, avoiding perfumed vaginal hygiene products and using water to wash the vulvo-vaginal area. Research has shown an association between phytoestrogens and modest improvements to vaginal dryness, so including soy products in your diet may help too. Maintaining a healthy vaginal ecosystem can help too.

Some helpful websites and resources:

Australasian Menopause Society

www.menopause.org.au

Jean Hailes for Women's Health

https://www.jeanhailes.org.au/health-a-z/vulva-vagina-ovaries-uterus/vulva-vaginal-irritation and https://assets.jeanhailes.org.au/Booklets/The_vulva.pdf

North American Menopause Society

www.menopause.org

International Menopause Society

www.imsociety.org

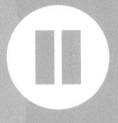

Chapter 11
LOW LIBIDO

Yesterday is history, tomorrow a mystery ...

Just as day turns into night and the sun rises and falls, the same could be said for one's libido. Reliable, predictable, expected, dependable, a never-ending quality. On call and available to turn on in an instant. Needless to say, I've enjoyed a healthy, active, sex life with 'sexy time' being a favourite pastime, thanks to my high sex-drive and stamina.

As I write this book, I contemplate how naive I've been to think that my libido was another characteristic of my personality that was constant. A natural personal resource that allowed performance on cue at the click of a finger – how wrong I've been.

What was once an amusement high on my list of priorities has fallen to the bottom. My sexual desires are less frequent and it's not from a lack of trying. Although that's the depressing part, I never had to try in the past to be turned on, I was on 24/7.

Imagine a V8 supercharged performance car: sleek, fast, exhilarating, powerful, dependable, the ultimate dream machine. Now consider this an old Kombi: slow, heavy, sluggish, it's often hard to start, conks out regularly and runs out of puff halfway up the hill.

Sexually I've always been comfortable in my own skin, but foreplay can now be tedious, orgasms elusive, and sexy time incredibly frustrating. A lovemaking session has become hard work and exhausting for my very patient, over-accommodating, considerate husband. I'm quick to give in and admit defeat, but not my man, who has great staying power and is determined to see the job completed to satisfaction.

Needless to say, things are really changing, and now I'm not so on, I am trying to determine what's added to the demise of my sex life. What comes first: the chicken or the egg? Does the pain associated with a dry vagina impact my libido or does my lack of libido stop the downstairs from juicing up? The crazy sexual desires that were once innate are few and far between. Sadly, my husband is also having to adjust to not having his 'horn bag' of a wife that he's cherished for 35 years!

It's clear to say my V8 supercar is adrift, with a GPS that's heading in a new direction – down a path of possible self-destruction, toward the couch where a hot cup of tea, a bickie and Netflix series awaits!

Yesterday was history, tomorrow a mystery, and whilst I continue to navigate this perimenopause journey, I know I need to focus on the present, let go of the past and appreciate a good cuppa – such is life!

Dear Dr Rosie,

This is a talk I would much prefer to avoid — I could Google 'dry vagina' but don't want it popping up in my news feed, so I hope you have all the answers!

- I'd really like to know what came first, the chicken or the egg — the dry vagina or the lack of libido?!
- What happened to the multiple orgasms and randy thoughts?
- Is it all in my head, or could my changing body shape be impacting my sex drive?

Thanks,
Jo

Let's talk about low libido

Hi Jo,

You wondered which comes first: the chicken or the egg; the dry vagina or the lack of libido. The short answer is, "It's complicated." You may have gathered by now that the answer is not a simple A leads to B; yes, the answer is more that it's the result of a combination of things. In a moment I will share with you the parable of the washing machine but before that let's talk about libido.

Libido and sexual arousal

When we talk about libido and sexual arousal, they sound the same thing; however, they are a little bit different. Libido is that primal physical sexual urge, that baseline interest in sex. Sexual arousal is the anticipatory excitement in mind and body, the increased blood flow to female nipples, clitoris, and vagina, and lubrication preparing for sexual intercourse. Let me reassure you that there is a wide range of normal. For example, Emma (not her real name) shared how she absolutely adores her partner but said, "If I have a choice between getting a good night's sleep and getting it on with my partner, sleep wins out every time. At the end of my day, all I want to do is crawl into bed and close my eyes." In contrast, let's call her Simone, is ready, willing and able and feels frustrated that her partner "doesn't show any interest whatsoever."

It is said that the largest sexual organ is our brain and sexual desire involves the intimacy of trust, love, connection and communication. For example, let's call her Beth, says: "My concerns about my partner's health issues initially resulted in a blip in the way we express our sexual intimacy. At first, I didn't feel so much in the way of physical desire and I had trouble relaxing because I was worried how getting intimate might affect him. After our blip, we discovered some other ways to express our love and desire for each other. We have had to change the way we previously physically did things; however, it works for both of us and now we both find it deeply satisfying."

The parable of the washing machine

I have a washing machine that functions brilliantly every time. I put the clothes in, dial up the appropriate wash cycle, press the start button and ... voila! A beautiful wash every time. However, before I can do all that, I have to enter a relatively simple three-digit code and if I don't enter the code correctly then no amount of my pleading, cajoling and threats moves my washing machine to perform. And in a funny life-imitates-art irony (let's call those old jokes about men's ability to do the laundry 'art' for the moment), if I ask my husband to do the laundry, it doesn't matter whether I write the instructions down or not, or how detailed they are, the fact is that my washing machine just simply won't 'perform' at random times, especially if he's trying to rush it!

I compare the three buttons to three big areas of lives: our *physical, mental/emotional* and *social* functioning. For our libido to get juiced up ready to go, programmed and be functioning, all three of them – the physical, mental/emotional and social areas of our life – usually need to be aligned.

The physical button

From a purely physical perspective, perimenopausal women tend to have an issue with vaginal dryness in terms of insufficient sexual arousal and lubrication rather than the low oestrogen level that comes after the final menstrual period and carries through menopause. Remember, during perimenopause oestrogen levels fluctuate erratically; sometimes oestrogen levels are high, accompanied by breast discomfort and fluid retention and at other times, low oestrogen levels can lead to hot flushes, sleep disruption and vaginal dryness. When you are in the low-oestrogen vaginal dryness state, then friction even from what has been a previously pleasurable source can feel more like sandpaper, and so understandably intercourse can feel sore or painful. However, there may be other underlying physical medical conditions: iron deficiency, anaemia, under-functioning thyroid, or painful parts – arthritis, sore hips, low-back pain. Several common medications such as antidepressants, antihypertensives for elevated blood pressure, antipsychotics, and antiepileptics can also contribute to a low libido. If in doubt, check it out and have a chat to your doctor about other treatment options that may be available.

It can be difficult for both intimate partners. Lack of understanding about what is happening, not wanting to talk about the issue and embarrassment can so easily come about from lack of communication. As we have previously seen, concerns about our partner's health issues may also contribute to the mix.

The mental button

Jo, you asked about what had happened to your multiple orgasms and randy thoughts. There are a few different things that might be happening here. Depression, anxiety, worries about family, workplace or financial concerns, low self-esteem, concerns about body image, or previous sexual or physical abuse can all turn down the enthusiasm for sex. And then there is the trust issue. If our intimate partner has betrayed our trust then it takes time to rebuild that trust (if ever) and they need to understand that there is no hurrying that.

A 49-years-wise lady, let's call her Kerry, was emerging from 18 months of breast cancer treatment, still grieving the recent death of her beloved mother and was wrestling with guilt because she made excuses to avoid having sex with her, as she put it, "long-suffering" partner. Basically, when men or women expend their energy on meeting the demands of day-to-day life, there may not be much energy left in the tank and crashing into bed to sleep may be much more desirable than a rumble. This applies to men too, and let's face it, having our partner at least seem *interested* is going to do more for our own libidos than if they get into bed and only ever turn out the light.

But what about how you feel about yourself? Is it all in your head or could your changing body shape be impacting your sex drive? You may remember that we talked about how our thoughts, feelings and behaviours are all interrelated, as seen in the following diagram.

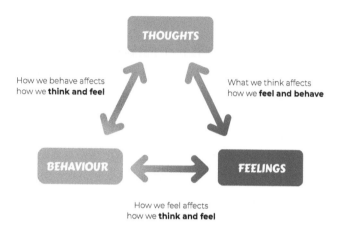

You are correct Jo, that our body confidence and the way we feel about our changing body shape can influence our sexual appetite. OK, so our body is changing and be more of a Babushka than a Barbie. How about we start giving ourselves a break and be kinder and gentler with ourselves? How about we stop comparing ourselves to others and stop find ourselves wanting? How about we start accepting our body, appreciating our health and celebrating our curves?

The social button

The social button may include a lack of opportunity. At this age and stage in life, many of us are facing having teenage or adult children still living at home, or even parents having to stay with us for extended periods. Some adult children have moved back home whilst transitioning from one place to another, and some stay on for a long time due to study commitments.

Tina (not her real name), who at 46 has two young teen-agers in the house, says that she freezes whenever something amorous starts to happen. "I am so worried that someone is going to walk in on us. Their bedroom is right next to ours; the walls are paper-thin and if we put a lock on the bedroom door and it is shut, then they are definitely going to know what is happening."

The point is, finding time, dealing with the discomfort and addressing any embarrassment or mental issues may seem challenging, but it is probably easier than you might imagine, with a little ingenuity.

Jo, with so many changes happening at this transitioning stage of life, it is not uncommon for a woman to feel changes in the experience of her own sensuality and changes in her sexual desire, arousal and activity. It is not uncommon for a woman to continue to be physically engaged in a sexually intimate relationship and yet feel great distress in terms of emotional isolation. If you have, or anyone you know has, issues of concern in this area, then encourage them to talk with a doctor or a counsellor they feel comfortable with to discuss this important aspect of their life.

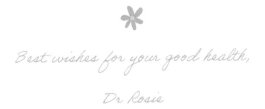

Best wishes for your good health,

Dr Rosie

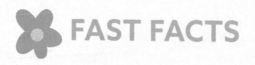# FAST FACTS

Which comes first: the chicken or the egg; the dry vagina or the lack of libido?

The short answer is, "It's complicated," and you may have gathered by now that the answer is not a simple A leads to B; yes, the answer is more the result of a combination of things. I compare the three buttons to three big areas of lives: our *physical*, *mental/emotional* and *social* functioning.

Physical:

Low oestrogen levels can result in vaginal dryness, and then friction even from what has been a previously pleasurable source can feel more like sandpaper, and so understandably intercourse can feel sore or painful.

However, underlying physical medical conditions or side effects of some common medications can also contribute to a low libido. If in doubt, have a chat to your doctor about other treatment options that may be available.

Mental:

Depression, anxiety, worries about family, workplace or financial concerns, low self-esteem, concerns about body image, and previous sexual or physical abuse can all turn down the enthusiasm for sex.

Social:

This may include a lack of opportunity. At this age and stage in life, many of us are facing having teenage or adult children still living at home, or even parents having to stay with us for extended periods. Finding time, dealing with the discomfort, and addressing any embarrassment or mental issues may seem challenging – but is probably easier than you might imagine, with a little ingenuity.

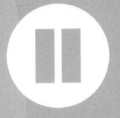

Chapter 12
THE WATERWORKS

Being pissed off

I believe that there is a direct correlation between physical and emotional health and wellbeing. Therefore, what is going on in our mind impacts what's happening in the body. Have you ever considered that maybe there really is a lot more going on than just a sore back, a wonky knee or a dodgy shoulder? Maybe our sore back is telling us we are unsupported and need propping up, our painful knee is instinctively saying that we're heading in the wrong direction in life, and our aching shoulder is clearly telling us to lighten the load and not carry the weight of the world on our shoulders.

Considering I'm now needing to wee more than ever, it's obviously something that is really pissing me off! Well, there's no surprise that this perimenopause state is enough to piss any woman off. On my last six-hour flight I needed to urinate five times. I now monitor my fluid intake around appointments and I've discovered all the public facilities in the region to avoid having to ask clients to use their toilet. Getting up and down through the night with a bursting bladder reminds me of being pregnant all over again, though I'm fortunate to not suffer from urinary tract infections (UTIs) like many of my friends. They express that UTIs are reoccurring and very debilitating; some struggled with UTIs as a younger woman whilst others have never experienced a UTI until peri-menopause. They describe how the insides of their vaginas sting and feel paper thin; plus the friction from intercourse leaves them raw, tender, inflamed and very uncomfortable. The thought of intercourse makes them cringe and therefore they avoid 'sexy time' at all costs even though some of them have raised libidos and want heaps of sex! With the added burning pain and discomfort associated with urination, they are irritated, frustrated and obviously very pissed off!

How ironic that UTIs are common in young women from having too much sex and now, in middle age and peri-menopause, UTIs prevent you from having sex!

My girlfriend tells a story of her mother visiting her GP with recurring UTIs during menopause. Her male physician explained with much conviction that women were badly designed, as God created the playground too close to the sewage works – WTF!

My theory behind 'for every physical there's an emotional' doesn't ring true when hormones are involved. I guess hormonal changes increase our risks of UTIs and I wonder if we can blame hormones for every other perceived issue that we are experiencing at this time. It surprises me constantly how rapidly my body is changing – from day to day, from my head down to my toes, from my inside to my outside.

Dear Dr Rosie,

- What's with the overactive bladder?
- Are urinary tract infections more common with perimenopause, and if so, why?
- What are your thoughts on the 'playground being too close to the sewage works'?

Thanks,
Jo

Let's talk about the waterworks

You mentioned being 'pissed off' and I am glad that you did because many women tend to suffer in silence with urinary issues. Every day, women with waterworks worries wear a track back and forth to the nearest bathroom. There are many bleary-eyed women who empty their bladder before going to bed and are still getting up to urinate two, three or four times during the night. In medical-speak, getting up to urinate at night is called *nocturia*. And according to a Californian study[1], nocturia is the most common bladder symptom that perimenopausal women experience, with around 7 out of 10 women having to get up at least once a night at least once a week.

You asked why you are experiencing an overactive bladder, and why your friends are experiencing more frequent urinary tract infections (UTIs). And whilst we are discussing bladder issues, I thought we should also look at urinary incontinence: those 'whoops!' moments when we cough, sneeze, jog or do star jumps. Let's start with the overactive bladder.

Overactive bladder

An overactive bladder is about irritability and urgency, needing to urinate frequently, which means more than eight times over 24 hours, having to go when you need to go, and getting up more than once to use the bathroom at night.

Our bladder has two jobs: storing and emptying urine. Normally the bladder wall muscle relaxes and allows the bladder to stretch and fill like a balloon. However, if the bladder wall muscle is irritated, it contracts to squeeze and empty the bladder before it is full. When this happens, a woman may experience a frequent and urgent need to pass urine (although the amount may be small), which can be accompanied by accidental uncontrollable leakage. A vaginal delivery, chronic constipation, being an unhealthy weight and older age can predispose us to this condition.

Is there any self-help for an overactive bladder?

I remember the travel details of one anxious lady, let's call her Sue, with overactive bladder. There were the two to three 'just-in-case' toilet stops before getting on the plane, requesting the seat allocation near the rear of the plane for quick toilet access, her trip to the loo before landing and then the one on the way to the baggage carousel. Her partner was pissed off, to say the least, and arguments sometimes ensued. Thankfully, a few lifestyle and behavioural modifications settled her symptoms and curtailed the crankiness.

There are several lifestyle changes which have been shown to be effective and worth a try to help manage an overactive bladder.

Consider limiting your consumption of caffeine. Caffeine has a mild diuretic effect and a stimulatory effect on the bladder wall muscle. You may find that reducing or avoiding caffeinated beverages including coffee and energy drinks helps reduce the symptoms of an overactive bladder.

You can also try bladder retraining to help your bladder hold more urine and decrease the number of times you need to head to the toilet. There are two parts to this technique. First, you start with a schedule of going to the toilet at specific short set times during the day. If you need feel the need to go the toilet before one of these timed visits, you practise what is called the 'Freeze and Squeeze' technique when the sense of urgency arises. The 'Freeze and Squeeze' technique involves pelvic floor strengthening exercises. As your bladder control improves, delay the time of your scheduled visit to the toilet by 15 minutes. The goal is to increase your time intervals between toilet trips to a normal three to four hours during the daytime and once at night.

Stopping smoking is also an important step because many smokers not only develop a chronic cough, which can put a lot of strain on the pelvic floor muscles and make stress incontinence worse, but also cigarette smoke is an irritant to the bladder that increases the symptoms of an overactive bladder. Further, smoking is a risk factor for developing bladder cancer.

Pelvic floor muscles can be given a workout and strengthened with Kegel exercises which I will talk more about a bit later in this letter. A physiotherapist with expertise in women's pelvic health will help guide you here.

Avoid anything that will increase intra-abdominal pressure such as heavy lifting or straining with constipation. Drinking plenty of water, eating at least five serves of fibre-rich vegetables and two serves of fruit a day helps to normalise bowel movements to avoid straining with constipation which would place more pressure on the pelvic floor.

Maintain a healthy weight. Carrying too much weight, especially around the middle also puts pressure on the bladder.

If you find you are still having an issue, have a chat to your doctor about medications that may help.

Incontinence

Urge incontinence

I'm going to jump right in here and start the conversation about urinary incontinence because it is another one of those 'downstairs' issues that women tend not to talk about, not even with their doctor. In my experience, there are many perimenopausal women who feel anxious that they could have a 'whoops' moment. If you are having to get to the toilet urgently ('when you gotta go, you gotta go') or frequently ('here we go *again*') then you are most likely looking at an overactive bladder that can also be accompanied by leakage of urine. Urgently needing to urinate with accidental urine leakage is called *urge incontinence*.

Stress incontinence

Then there is the accidental leakage that can happen with a cough, sneeze, laugh or while lifting something heavy like an overfull shopping bag. This is known as *stress incontinence*.

The pelvic floor, as you can see from the following diagram, is a group of muscles located low down in the pelvis, like a hammock stretched from the tail bone at the back to the pubic bone in the front. The pelvic floor muscles support our internal organs of bladder, uterus and bowel to stay in the right place and contract (tighten) to give us control over when we urinate and defecate.

Female Pelvic Floor

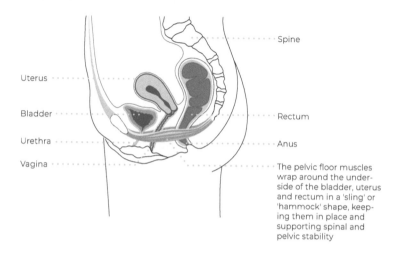

Uterus

Bladder

Urethra

Vagina

Spine

Rectum

Anus

The pelvic floor muscles wrap around the under-side of the bladder, uterus and rectum in a 'sling' or 'hammock' shape, keeping them in place and supporting spinal and pelvic stability

Being overweight, childbirth, and chronic constipation can all contribute to weakening the pelvic floor. When the pelvic floor muscles are weak, we are more likely to have less control over when we pass wind, faeces and urine. A weak pelvic floor can also result in the bladder, uterus or bowel dropping down further in the pelvis than is normal and this is called a *prolapse*. When we cough, laugh or sneeze, the pressure in our abdomen increases, pushing our bladder further down in the pelvis. If our pelvic floor muscles, which include the muscles that keep us from leaking urine, are weak, then abdominal pressure is greater than the bladder outlet muscles can manage, and this can result in accidental urine leakage.

Pelvic floor exercises

There is a lot of evidence that women who have stress incontinence will benefit from pelvic floor strengthening exercises, also commonly known as *Kegel exercises*. A review of data from 31 different trials involving 1817 women from 14 different countries found that pelvic floor muscle training can improve or even cure symptoms of stress urinary incontinence[2].

How can you know if you have strong or weak pelvic floor muscles? You can check for yourself. Next time you sit on the toilet, start to urinate and then see if you can stop the stream before you have completely emptied your bladder, then finish urinating (only try this once a week at most). You should feel the muscles in your vagina and anus tighten. This part of your pelvic floor controls bladder flow.

Now imagine you are trying to stop yourself from passing wind and squeeze the muscles around your anus (not your buttocks). This is the part of your pelvic floor that controls the rectum muscles.

Vaginal muscles can be tested by inserting your finger into the vagina and tightening as if you are stopping the flow of urine.

Information on how to perform Kegel exercises is widely available and there are specialist physiotherapists who can assess how well this area is functioning, teach correct pelvic exercise technique and help you monitor your progress.

If a prolapse is present, a vaginal pessary can be fitted by a doctor, pelvic floor physiotherapist, gynaecologist or urologist to support the bladder. This is a good option if surgery is not wanted. Alternatively, a pessary can provide short-term relief whilst waiting for surgery.

In Australia, the plight of incontinent women is taken seriously, so seriously that the National Women's Health Strategy 2020–2030[3] has detailed actions to improve treatment and support for both urinary and faecal incontinence in women.

Urinary tract infections

You've asked whether urinary tract infections are more common during perimenopause, but I want to first explain what they are, and why women are more prone to them than men. Urinary tract infection (UTI) is a general term to describe an infection anywhere in the urinary system. An infection in the bladder is called *cystitis*; an infection in the urethra is called *urethritis*; and an infection in the kidneys is called *pyelonephritis*. UTIs are most commonly caused by bacterial microorganisms.

Some of the symptoms of a UTI include:

- a burning or stinging sensation when passing urine
- feeling like you need to urinate frequently but only being able to pass a very small amount
- smelly or cloudy urine
- suprapubic pain, which is pain above the pubic bone.

If you think you have a urinary tract infection it is important that you see your doctor for assessment and treatment. Warning: if you are unwell with a high fever, low back or kidney pain, you may have a kidney infection, or if you have started taking antibiotics but have not felt any improvement, this is a potentially serious situation so do not delay. In this case, you are strongly advised to seek URGENT medical attention.

Why are UTIs common in women, and why are they more common during perimenopause?

Urinary tract infections are common in women, with one in two women developing a UTI at least once in their lifetime[4]. In Australia, one in three women will develop a UTI before the age of 24 (the lifetime risk for men is one in 20). There are several factors that predispose women to more frequent UTIs than men, which I will detail below.

Length of the urethra

One of the reasons why women are more prone to UTIs than men is that they have a shorter urethra, which makes it easier for bacteria to travel up into the bladder. The urethra is the tube passing from the bladder to the outside of the body. The female urethra is about four centimetres in length compared to the male urethra, which is 15 to 20 cm[5]. The female urethra is also straight, which makes it easier for *Escherichia coli* (commonly referred to as *E. coli*), which are bacteria that live in the bowel, to enter the urinary tract through the urethra. *E.coli* are the bacteria that most commonly cause UTIs.

Sexual intercourse

You may remember those younger years of pleasure and pain, with so-called 'honeymoon cystitis' following frequent intercourse. Sexual intercourse, a new sexual partner, and the use of diaphragms and spermicides all increase the risk of developing a UTI.

When there is a fraction too much friction, moisture is important. Ensure you take in plenty of oral fluids to maintain tissue hydration and apply a generous amount of a silicone-based preparation to lubricate and keep it comfortable. You may want to avoid spermicides on condoms and diaphragms as they can increase the risk of contracting a UTI. A number of studies have reported that spermicides containing nonoxynol-9 decrease the population of beneficial *Lactobacillus* species bacteria and encourages the colonisation by *E.coli*, so check the spermicide ingredients label.

Location, location, location

The close proximity of the anus to the vagina and urethra can result in bacteria tracking up the short urethra into the bladder and once they start to enjoy the warmth and stable pH of the bladder, they begin to multiply. Pre- and post-intercourse urination may reduce some of the spontaneity but helps flush away UTI-causing bacteria. And whilst you are on the loo you might want to check your positioning and timing. Correct positioning includes sitting comfortably on the toilet seat rather than hovering over it, as well as taking your time to ensure you have completely emptied your bladder. And when using toilet paper, remember to wipe from front to back to avoid sweeping bacteria from the anus toward the urethra.

Changing hormones

UTIs in women can also occur when hormones are changing. You may have experienced an UTI when your oestrogen level was lower before your period arrived. And remember those erratic fluctuations in oestrogen during the transitioning years I talked about earlier?

Declining oestrogen levels over the course of peri-menopause result in drier, thinner tissues, which makes the whole genital area more susceptible to friction, abrasions and infection. The lower oestrogen level also results in weakening of the muscles at the entrance to the urethra so they are not able to squeeze as tightly to close it off, which makes it easier for bacteria to travel up the short urethra and into the bladder. This is why UTIs may be more common as you pass through the perimenopause stage.

Are there any remedies for UTIs?

There is the option of taking a prophylactic antibiotic, which means taking a low-dose antibiotic daily or when you have intercourse. For many women who suffer with recurrent UTIs, this is helpful. When we talk about frequent or recurrent UTIs, it means more than two episodes in the last six months or more than three UTIs in the last 12 months. Best to have a discussion with your doctor about this.

With the issue of antibiotic resistance raising its head, a question is often raised about the benefit of cranberry juice, which is traditionally used in the prevention of UTIs. From laboratory studies there is evidence of cranberry's antibacterial, antifungal and antiadhesive properties; however, the evidence of the effectiveness of cranberry products in reducing the frequency or recurrence of UTIs is mixed.

A meta-analysis[6], of seven different randomised control studies, concluded: "Results suggest cranberry may be effective in preventing recurrent UTIs in generally healthy women, [and then the rider], however, larger high-quality studies are needed to confirm these findings."

The vaginal microbiome and acid–alkaline balance

The acid–alkaline balance in the vagina is important to maintain urogenital health. Lactic acid secreted by *Lactobacillus* species bacteria keeps the vagina at an acidic pH 4.0 to 5.0. When there are changes in the acid–alkaline balance in the vagina, this can be a signal for other types of bacteria to start overgrowing in the area. For example, the bacteria that cause bacterial vaginosis grow better in an alkaline environment of pH 7.0, producing a greyish or yellowish discharge with a fishy odour along with a burning and stinging sensation with urination. As a woman transitions through perimenopause, her declining oestrogen levels also lead to changes in the vaginal pH balance, and in turn a reduction of *Lactobacillus* flora-associated health. Low-dose vaginal oestrogen therapy has been shown to bring the pH back to a healthier range, increase *Lactobacillus* species abundance and help prevent UTIs from recurring.

The vaginal ecosystem is an area of ongoing study and more research is required to determine whether probiotics to modify the vaginal microbiome can reduce genitourinary symptoms. In the meantime, you could add probiotic foods containing 'good bacteria', such as fermented sauerkraut, kimchi and live-culture yoghurt, into your daily diet. However, a word to the wise. Whilst a little of what you like is beneficial, too much of a good thing is not always better. If you do want to start including fermented products into your diet, consider the adage to 'start low, go slow', otherwise you might end up with burping, bloating and abdominal discomfort.

Why is the playground located next to the sewage works?

Whilst we are talking about the vaginal microbiome, you asked why the playground is situated next to the sewage pipe? I recall one of my medical lecturers asking this same rhetorical question. Today, we have a better understanding as to why this might be the case. Research[7] has shown that early life events such as the mode of delivery affects the composition of the infant's gut microbiome. Due to the close proximity of the vagina and anus, babies born by vaginal delivery are exposed to organisms in the mother's gut biome. Many studies suggest that babies born by caesarean section have an infant gut microbiome which reflects the types of bacterial colonies found on their mother's skin compared with a child born by vaginal delivery who is exposed to their mother's vaginal, faecal and skin bacterial communities – bacteria that assist in the development of a healthy immune system and metabolism.

*

Jo, I hope you find this helpful.

Best wishes for your good health,

Dr Rosie

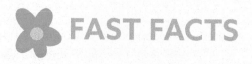 **FAST FACTS**

What is an overactive bladder?

An overactive bladder is about irritability and urgency, needing to urinate frequently, which means more than eight times over 24 hours, including having to get up more than once at night.

Incontinence

Urgent and frequent trips to the toilet can be accompanied by accidental leakage of urine, which is called *urge incontinence*.

The accidental leakage that may result from a cough, sneeze, laugh or lifting something heavy is known as *stress incontinence*.

Why are urinary tract infections (UTIs) common in women, and during perimenopause?

Urinary tract infections are common in women, with one in two women developing a UTI at least once in their lifetime. The *urethra* (the tube passing from the bladder to the outside of the body) in women is short and straight, making it easier for bacteria to be transferred from the bowel, which is near the urethra. Women are at increased risk of recurrent UTIs if they use a diaphragm or spermicide, if they have a new sexual partner or if have a tendency to constipation. Declining oestrogen levels can leave you more susceptible to UTIs, which is why they're often experienced before a menstrual period or during perimenopause.

Why is the playground located next to the sewage works?

Early life events such as the mode of delivery are important in establishing an infant's gut microbiome. Many studies suggest that babies born by caesarean section have an infant gut microbiome which reflects the types of bacterial colonies found on their mother's skin compared with a child born by vaginal delivery, who is exposed to their mother's vaginal, faecal and skin bacterial communities – bacteria that assist in the development of a healthy immune system and metabolism.

The golden ticket

My favourite movie as a child was *Charlie and the Chocolate Factory*. For those of you who are unfamiliar with the story, it's about obtaining an exclusive golden ticket for entry into Willy Wonka's Chocolate Factory. The golden ticket is hidden inside the wrapping of only five chocolate Wonka Bars. Inside the eccentric and reclusive Willy Wonka's magical factory exists a child's dream: a candy land, a river of chocolate, gummy bears, candy canes, chocolate and sweets.

Menopause Island is not dissimilar: a retreat where you will be totally indulged, the ultimate fantasy, exclusively for women who hold a golden ticket. A desert island where you will be pampered, indulged and waited on 24/7, but unfortunately not by short green Oompa-Loompas found only in fantasy chocolate factories!

On Menopause Island there are no responsibilities. You will not work, shop, clean, prepare meals, cook, or drive. Serving others, mobile phones and social media is not permitted on the island under any circumstances and will result in instant eviction. You will be required to undertake at least two body treatments per day. On offer are such delights as a full-body massage, facial, salt glow, body wrap, spa manicure and pedicure, and body scrub. Yoga, tai chi, meditation, relaxation and long beach walks are mandatory. You will have access to naturopathy, aromatherapy, reflexology, acupuncture, homeopathy, hypnotherapy, Ayurvedic and traditional medicine on demand.

To achieve a golden ticket, you MUST meet the following criteria:

- Have a vagina like a gravel pit
- Suffer from Middle Tyre Disease
- Be pissed off – often
- Be easily frustrated, irritated and deeply intolerant at times
- Be an expert at counting sheep
- Be happy, sad, happy, sad!
- Feel itchy-scratchy
- Your wardrobe is changing daily
- You are buying bigger handbags!
- You suffer from global warming – inside and outside

If you proudly possess at least five of the above attributes, you've arrived! Congratulations, your entry is free!

Menopause Island is a happy place, full of fun where you will feel level-headed, fully in control and not have a worry in the world. A place of total relaxation and indulgence, where you can rest, acknowledge your thoughts, take control of your emotions and be completely pampered. A sanctuary where you will feel safe and nurtured, and be provided with three hearty, wholesome meals per day.

There will be no frustrations or irritations on Menopause Island. You will sleep soundly for at least eight hours a night and will no longer be exhausted. You will have plenty of time to read all your unread books, including those you've been wanting to read for the past 20 years. You will enjoy catching up on journalling, scrapbooking, writing or sorting photos into albums – or you may choose to do absolutely nothing. You will be free to wear white jeans and pedal-pushers, or free-flowing, generous garments and elasticised pants for additional comfort if you prefer.

Menopause Island is a place to revisit your past, reset your future and finalise any unfinished business. A time to acknowledge your attributes, achievements, sacrifices and all your hard work raising a family. The perfect place to let go of the past and look forward to the future. You can embrace your curves, love your imperfections and worship yourself. A time to regroup, take stock and rewrite the next chapter in your book of life through wiser and brighter eyes.

Congratulations, you have made it! This is now the beginning of your third act – your wonder years.

The reality is, Menopause Island is not so much about being pampered and enjoying carefree scrapbooking time. Nevertheless, these are the years where we can choose to do a lot more of what we want to do, for ourselves, and to become more comfortable with who we are – inside our own skin. We can make fewer apologies for our intolerances and focus on our strengths, sharing our wisdom. Remember, in most cultures, the older woman is revered for her greying beauty, her *mana*, her ability to spread calm and nurture the wider families; she is a spokesperson for her tribe, and is consulted for her healing abilities.

We can think of these transitional years as being the time to find ourselves: who we are, why we are here, and what we wish to leave behind as our legacies; whether that's a family, a tribe, a garden, or relationships that are made better by our contributions to them. The journey we take to Menopause Island is therefore the time of discovery, and transition into becoming our real selves, if we allow ourselves to see this time as a positive part of our lives.

There may not be a candy land, gummy bears, candy canes or sweets on Menopause Island but one thing I can guarantee: there will be lots and lots of chocolate! For each of us, upon returning to our (real) lives we will be fulfilled, nourished, rested and grateful for the time that we have allowed ourselves to shine.

Dear Rosie,

I'm happy about there being a menopause Island in my fantasy on this transitional journey, and wish that there really were such places for us to ride out these challenging years in — for now, I guess I'll have to settle for weekends at the beach a few times a year, and raucous lunches with my girlfriends whenever we can all get together.

But Rosie, how does life look for us all beyond perimenopause?

Love Jo

Let's talk about 'and she lived healthily ever after'

Dear Jo,

I like the sound of Menopause Island, a personal space or a physical place to relax, reflect and rejuvenate.

Pause.
Take a 'time out' breath.

I say this with compassion because so many midlife women have shared with me that one of the biggest challenges they face is how to find balance in their life whilst dealing with the stress served up by several different life events: how to balance their work-life commitments, the changing dynamics in their family, their relationships, ensuring they have financial security, how do they cope with loss and grief, and where are they ever going to find time to rediscover who they are?

How about we consider this 'pause as an opportunity: a time to ensure that we are fit for the menopause, rocking and ready to enjoy the next chapter of our lives.

If we hold to the knowledge that we have within us the power to write and create our own story, then we have within us the power to make changes in our lives that will support our health and wellbeing. That change is a gift. Whether you know it or not, the lifestyle choices you make today are setting you up for your years ahead. Let's ensure your life adventure reads '... and she lived healthfully ever after'.

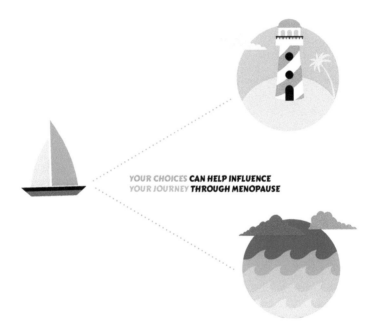

YOUR CHOICES **CAN HELP INFLUENCE** YOUR JOURNEY **THROUGH MENOPAUSE**

In a way, we can liken this perimenopause phase to childbirth. Childbirth is natural; it is not a disease. Childbirth is the transition process from pregnancy to holding an infant in your arms. Each childbirth is a personal experience with a lot of hormonal changes, together with a lot of strong physical and emotional changes that can happen too. Every woman who lives long enough to move through this will birth herself into what is potentially the most powerful phase of her life.

Jo, thank you for asking so many wonderful questions about your journey towards menopause.

Best wishes for your good health,

Dr Rosie

Acknowledgements

I am so grateful and acknowledge the following people for assisting me on this journey.

Firstly, to my co-author Joanne Vines, who shared her secrets and wicked sense of humour over numerous cups of chai tea.

To Sam Wardman and Kate Amos for encouraging us to 'go for it' over dinner one night.

The 'Word Witch', Dixie Carlton, who helped me unpack what was in my head and coached, cajoled and encouraged me throughout the writing of this book.

The 'Conveyer of Calm', Ann Wilson, and all at Indie Experts, for transforming my notes into a book.

And my ever patient and encouraging husband Alex, who has been a constant support from the beginning.

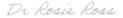

Dr Rosie Ross

My sincere thanks and gratitude to:

Pryde, my gorgeous, adorable, supportive and loving husband. Thank you for allowing me to be me, and for sharing my vagina with the world!

Dr Rosie, my intelligent, funny, co-writer friend and GP. I have loved every moment of this journey with you. Thank you for your brilliance and therapy along the way.

Karen, my beautiful gentle friend and sister from another mother! Thank you for your ear, wittiness, humour, and sharing parts of yourself that have been included in this book; I'm sincerely grateful.

Sam and Kate, this book is for you for when the time comes. Thank you for supporting Rosie and I through this project, we are forever thankful.

My mum Julee, dad Sam, sister Tina and brothers Charles and Anthony, thank you for the memories and stories that have made this book. I am truly grateful for my wonderful childhood and the woman I've become.

Ngahine and Zak, my children whom I love and adore. Sorry if I've been irrational, intolerant, snappy and moody; oh well, shit happens!

To the beautiful women in my life who have shared their stories and contributed in some way: Janice, Kay, Cher, Kate, Lou, Carol, Sharon, Piere, Julie, Tracey, Nell, Karen, Michelle, Megan, Ange, Jacqui & Vyvienne. Thank you for your friendship and your honesty.

Joanne Vines

Endnotes

Chapter 1

1 Prior, J. (1998). Perimenopause: The complex endocrinology of the menopausal transition. *Endocrine Reviews, 19*(4), 397–428.

2 Mihm, M., Gangooly, S., & Muttukrishna, S. (2011). The normal menstrual cycle in women. *Animal reproduction science, 124*(3–4), 229–236.

3 Bull, J. R., Rowland, S. P., Scherwitzl, E. B., Scherwitzl, R., Danielsson, K. G., & Harper, J. (2019). Real-world menstrual cycle characteristics of more than 600,000 menstrual cycles. *NPJ Digital Medicine, 2,* 83.

4 Harlow, S. D., Mitchell, E. S., Crawford, S., Nan, B., Little, R., Taffe, J., & ReSTAGE Collaboration (2008). The ReSTAGE Collaboration: Defining optimal bleeding criteria for onset of early menopausal transition. *Fertility and Sterility, 89*(1), 129–140.

5 McKinlay, S. M., Brambilla, D. J., & Posner, J. G. (1992). The normal menopause transition. *Maturitas, 14*(2), 103–115.

6 Harlow, S. D., & Paramsothy, P. (2011). Menstruation and the menopausal transition. *Obstetrics and Gynecology Clinics of North America, 38*(3), 595–607.

7 Biela, U. (2002). Czynniki determinujace wiek naturalnej menopauzy [Determinants of the age at natural menopause]. *Przeglad Lekarski, 59*(3), 165–169.

Chapter 3

1 Karvonen-Gutierrez, C., & Kim, C. (2016). Association of mid-life changes in body size, body composition and obesity status with the menopausal transition. *Healthcare, 4*(3), 42.

2 Women's Health Australia. (2017). *1946–51 Cohort, Summary 1996–2016.* Retrieved from http://www.alswh.org.au/images/content/pdf/Cohort _summaries/1946-51%20Cohort%20Summary%201996-2016.pdf

3   Sternfeld, B., Wang, H., Quesenberry, C., Adams, B., Everson-Rose, S., & Greendale, G., Matthews, K. A., Torrens, J. I., & Sowers, M. (2004). Physical activity and changes in weight and waist circumference in midlife women: Findings from the Study of Women's Health Across the Nation. *American Journal of Epidemiology*, *160*(9), 912–922.

4   Ambikairajah, A., Walsh, E., Tabatabaei-Jafari, H., & Cherbuin, N. (2019). Fat mass changes during menopause: A metaanalysis. *American Journal of Obstetrics and Gynecology*, *221*(5), 393–409.e50.

5   Franklin, R. M., Ploutz-Snyder, L., & Kanaley, J. A. (2009). Longitudinal changes in abdominal fat distribution with menopause. *Metabolism: Clinical and Experimental*, *58*(3), 311–315.

6   Davis, S. R., Castelo-Branco, C., Chedraui, P., Lumsden, M. A., Nappi, R. E., Shah, D., Villaseca, P., & Writing Group of the International Menopause Society for World Menopause Day 2012. (2012). Understanding weight gain at menopause. *Climacteric: The Journal of the International Menopause Society*, *15*(5), 419–429.

7   Sowers, M., Zheng, H., Tomey, K., Karvonen-Gutierrez, C., Jannausch, M., Li, X., Yosef, M., & Symons, J. (2007). Changes in body composition in women over six years at midlife: Ovarian and chronological aging. *The Journal of Clinical Endocrinology and Metabolism*, *92*(3), 895–901.

8   Pi-Sunyer X. (2009). The medical risks of obesity. *Postgraduate Medicine*, *121*(6), 21–33.

9   Paley, C., & Johnson, M. (2018). Abdominal obesity and metabolic syndrome: Exercise as medicine? *BMC Sports Science, Medicine and Rehabilitation*, *10*(1).

10 Freemantle, N., Holmes, J., Hockey, A., & Kumar, S. (2008). How strong is the association between abdominal obesity and the incidence of type 2 diabetes? *International Journal of Clinical Practice*, *62*(9), 1391–1396.

11 Kanaya, A. M., Vittinghoff, E., Shlipak, M. G., Resnick, H. E., Visser, M., Grady, D., & BarrettConnor, E. (2003). Association of total and central obesity with mortality in postmenopausal women with coronary heart disease. *American Journal of Epidemiology*, *158*(12), 1161–1170.

12 Smitka, K., & Marešová, D. (2015). Adipose tissue as an endocrine organ: an update on pro-inflammatory and anti-inflammatory microenvironment. *Prague Medical Report*, *116*(2), 87–111.

13 Misra, A., Wasir J. S., & Vikram, N. K. (2005). Waist circumference criteria for the diagnosis of abdominal obesity are not applicable uniformly to all populations and ethnic groups. *Nutrition*, *21*(9), 969–76.

14 Harris, M. F. (2013). The metabolic syndrome. *Australian Family Physicians*, *42*(8), 524–527.

15 Department of Health. (2014). *Fact sheet – How much sugar is in what we drink?* Canberra: Commonwealth of Australia. Retrieved from https://

www1.health.gov.au/internet/publications/publishing.nsf/Content/
sugar-drinks-toc~sugar-drinks-3-fact-sheets~sugar-drinks-factsheet-
3-3-sugar-what-drink

16 Department of Health. (2019). *Standard drinks guide*. Canberra:
    Commonwealth of Australia. Retrieved from health.gov.au/health-
    topics/alcohol/about-alcohol/standard-drinks-guide

17 Yeomans, M. R. (2010). Alcohol, appetite and energy balance: Is alcohol
    intake a risk factor for obesity? *Physiology & Behavior, 100*(1), 82–89.

18 World Cancer Research Fund. (2020). *Alcoholic drinks: Alcoholic
    drinks and the risk of cancer*. Retrieved from https://www.wcrf.org/
    dietandcancer/exposures/alcoholic-drinks

19 Australian Bureau of Statistics. (2018). *Fruit and vegetable consumption*.
    Canberra. Retrieved from https://www.abs.gov.au/ausstats/abs@.
    nsf/Lookup/by%20Subject/4364.0.55.001~2017-18~Main%20
    Features~Fruit%20and%20vegetable%20consumption~105

20 Ge, L., Sadeghirad, B., Ball, G., da Costa, B. R., Hitchcock, C. L., Svendrovski,
    A., Kiflen, R., Quadri, K., Kwon, H. Y., Karamouzian, M., Adams-Webber,
    T., Ahmed, W., Damanhoury, S., Zeraatkar, D., Nikolakopoulou, A.,
    Tsuyuki, R. T., Tian, J., Yang, K., Guyatt, G. H., & Johnston, B. C. (2020).
    Comparison of dietary macronutrient patterns of 14 popular named
    dietary programmes for weight and cardiovascular risk factor reduction
    in adults: Systematic review and network meta-analysis of randomised
    trials. *BMJ, 369*, m696.

21 Department of Health. (2014). *Make your move – Sit less, be active
    for life!* Canberra: Commonwealth of Australia. Retrieved from
    https://www1.health.gov.au/internet/main/publishing.nsf/content/
    F01F92328EDADA5BCA257BF0001E720D/$File/brochure%20PA%20
    Guidelines_A5_18-64yrs.PDF.

22 Buettner, D. (2010). *The Blue Zones*. Washington, D.C.: National
    Geographic Society.

23 Painter, S. L., Ahmed, R., Hill, J. O., Kushner, R. F., Lindquist, R., Brunning,
    S., & Margulies, A. (2017). What matters in weight loss? An in-depth analysis
    of self-monitoring. *Journal of Medical Internet Research, 19*(5), e160.

24 Dalle Grave, R., Sartirana, M., & Calugi, S. (2020). Personalized cognitive-
    behavioural therapy for obesity (CBT-OB): Theory, strategies and
    procedures. *BioPsychoSocial Medicine, 14*, 5. doi: 10.1186/s13030-020-
    00177-9

Chapter 4

1   Born, L., Koren, G., Lin, E., & Steiner, M. (2008). A new, female-specific
    irritability rating scale. *Journal of Psychiatry & Neuroscience, 33*(4),
    344–354.

2   Behl, C. (2002). Oestrogen as a neuroprotective hormone. *Nature Reviews. Neuroscience, 3*(6), 433–442.

3   Santoro, N., & Randolph, J. F., Jr. (2011). Reproductive hormones and the menopause transition. *Obstetrics and Gynecology Clinics of North America, 38*(3), 455–466.

4   Gordon, J. L., Rubinow, D. R., Eisenlohr-Moul, T. A., Xia, K., Schmidt, P. J., & Girdler, S. S. (2018). Efficacy of transdermal estradiol and micronized progesterone in the prevention of depressive symptoms in the menopause transition: A randomized clinical trial. *JAMA Psychiatry, 75*(2), 149–157.

5   Hale, G. E., Hughes, C. L., Burger, H. G., Robertson, D. M., & Fraser, I. S. (2009). Atypical estradiol secretion and ovulation patterns caused by luteal out-of-phase (LOOP) events underlying irregular ovulatory menstrual cycles in the menopausal transition. *Menopause, 16*(1), 50–59.

6   Raglan, G. B., Schulkin, J., Juliano, L. M., & Micks, E. A. (2020). Obstetrician-gynecologists' screening and management of depression during perimenopause. *Menopause, 27*(4), 393–397.

7   Enjezab, B., Zarehosseinabadi, M., Farzinrad, B., & Dehghani, A. (2019). The effect of mindfulness-based cognitive therapy on quality of life in perimenopausal women. *Iranian Journal of Psychiatry and Behavioral Sciences, 13*(1): e86525. doi: 10.5812/ijpbs.86525

8   World Health Organization. (1946). Preamble to the Constitution of the World Health Organization as adopted by the International Health Conference, New York, 19–22 June, 1946. New York: World Health Organization.

9   Kuhlman, K. R., Robles, T. F., Dooley, L. N., Boyle, C. C., Haydon, M. D., & Bower, J. E. (2018). Within-subject associations between inflammation and features of depression: Using the flu vaccine as a mild inflammatory stimulus. *Brain, Behavior, and Immunity, 69*, 540–547.

10 Amodeo, G.,Trusso, M. A., & Fagiolini, A. (2017). Depression and inflammation: Disentangling a clear yet complex and multifaceted link. *Neuropsychiatry, 7*(4). doi:10.4172/NEUROPSYCHIATRY.1000236

11 Karaoulanis, S. E., Daponte, A., Rizouli, K. A., Rizoulis, A. A., Lialios, G. A., Theodoridou, C. T., Christakopoulos, C., & Angelopoulos, N. V. (2012). The role of cytokines and hot flashes in perimenopausal depression. *Annals of General Psychiatry, 11*, 9.

12 Guo, L., Ren, L., & Zhang, C. (2018). Relationship between depression and inflammatory factors and brain-derived neurotrophic factor in patients with perimenopause syndrome. *Experimental and Therapeutic Medicine, 15*(5), 4436–4440.

13 Spedding, S. (2014). Vitamin D and depression: A systematic review and meta-analysis comparing studies with and without biological flaws. *Nutrients, 6*(4), 1501–1518.

14 Taren, A. A., Gianaros, P. J., Greco, C. M., Lindsay, E. K., Fairgrieve, A., Brown, K. W., Rosen, R. K., Ferris, J. L., Julson, E., Marsland, A. L., Bursley, J. K., Ramsburg, J., & Creswell, J. D. (2015). Mindfulness meditation training alters stress-related amygdala resting state functional connectivity: A randomized controlled trial. *Social Cognitive and Affective Neuroscience*, *10*(12), 1758–1768.

15 Kwak, S., Lee, T. Y., Jung, W. H., Hur, J. W., Bae, D., Hwang, W. J., Cho, K., Lim, K. O., Kim, S. Y., Park, H. Y., & Kwon, J. S. (2019). The immediate and sustained positive effects of meditation on resilience are mediated by changes in the resting brain. *Frontiers in Human Neuroscience*, *13*, 101.

16 Nayak, G., Kamath, A., Kumar, P. N., & Rao, A. (2014). Effect of yoga therapy on physical and psychological quality of life of perimenopausal women in selected coastal areas of Karnataka, India. *Journal of Mid-Life Health*, *5*(4), 180–185.

17 Vaze, N., & Joshi, S. (2010). Yoga and menopausal transition. *Journal of Mid-Life Health*, *1*(2), 56–58.

18 Innes, K. E., Selfe, T. K., & Taylor, A. G. (2008). Menopause, the metabolic syndrome, and mind-body therapies. *Menopause*, *15*(5), 1005–1013.

19 Russo, M. A., Santarelli, D. M., & O'Rourke, D. (2017). The physiological effects of slow breathing in the healthy human. *Breathe*, *13*(4), 298–309.

20 Ma, X., Yue, Z. Q., Gong, Z. Q., Zhang, H., Duan, N. Y., Shi, Y. T., Wei, G. X., & Li, Y. F. (2017). The effect of diaphragmatic breathing on attention, negative affect and stress in healthy adults. *Frontiers in Psychology*, *8*, 874.

Chapter 5

1 Brown, T., & Krishnamurthy, K. (2018). Histology, Dermis [Ebook]. Treasure Island (FL): StatPearls Publishing.

2 Liu, F., Hamer, M., Deelen, J., Lall, J., Jacobs, L., & van Heemst, D., Murray, P. G., Wollstein, A., de Craen, A. J., Uh, H. W., Zeng, C., Hofman, A., Uitterlinden, A. G., Houwing-Duistermaat, J. J., Pardo, L. M., Beekman, M., Slagboom, P. E., Nijsten, T., Kayser, M., & Gunn, D. A. (2016). The MC1R Gene and Youthful Looks. *Current Biology*, *26*(9), 1213–1220. doi. org/10.1016/j.cub.2016.03.008

3 Wilkinson, H. N., & Hardman, M. J. (2017). The role of estrogen in cutaneous ageing and repair. *Maturitas*, *103*, 60–64.

4 Calleja-Agius, J., Brincat, M., & Borg, M. (2013). Skin connective tissue and ageing. *Best Practice & Research: Clinical Obstetrics & Gynaecology*, *27*(5), 727–740.

5 Nair, P. (2014). Dermatosis associated with menopause. *Journal of Mid-Life Health*, *5*(4), 168–175.

6 Flament, F., Bazin, R., Rubert, V., Simonpietri, E., Piot, B., & Laquieze, S. (2013). Effect of the sun on visible clinical signs of aging in Caucasian skin. *Clinical, Cosmetic and Investigational Dermatology*, *6*, 221–232.

7   Goodman, G., Armour, K., Kolodziejczyk, J., Santangelo, S., & Gallagher, C. (2018). Comparison of self-reported signs of facial ageing among Caucasian women in Australia versus those in the USA, the UK and Canada. *Australasian Journal of Dermatology, 59*(2), 108–117.

8   Cancer Council Australia. (2020). Skin cancer. Retrieved from https://www.cancer.org.au/about-cancer/types-of-cancer/skin-cancer.html

9   Matsui, M., Pelle, E., Dong, K., & Pernodet, N. (2016). Biological rhythms in the skin. *International Journal of Molecular Sciences, 17*(6), 801.

10 Australian Sleep Health Foundation. (2020). Sleep needs across the lifespan. Retrieved from https://www.sleephealthfoundation.org.au/files/pdfs/Sleep-Needs-Across-Lifespan.pdf

11 DermNet NZ. (2020). Smoking and its effects on the skin. Retrieved from https://dermnetnz.org/topics/smoking-and-its-effects-on-the-skin/

12 Urbańska, M., Nowak, G., & Florek, E. (2012). Wpływ palenia tytoniu na starzenie sie skóry [Cigarette smoking and its influence on skin aging]. *Przeglad Lekarski, 69*(10), 1111–1114.

13 Goodman, G. D., Kaufman, J., Day, D., Weiss, R., Kawata, A. K., Garcia, J. K., Santangelo, S., & Gallagher, C. J. (2019). Impact of smoking and alcohol use on facial aging in women: Results of a large multinational, multiracial, cross-sectional survey. *The Journal of Clinical and Aesthetic Dermatology, 12*(8), 28–39.

14 Palma, L., Tavares Marques, L., Bujan, J., & Monteiro Rodrigues, L. (2015). Dietary water affects human skin hydration and biomechanics. *Clinical, Cosmetic and Investigational Dermatology, 8*, 413–21.

15 Purnamawati, S., Indrastuti, N., Danarti, R., & Saefudin, T. (2017). The role of moisturizers in addressing various kinds of dermatitis: A review. *Clinical Medicine & Research, 15*(3-4), 75–87.

16 Lodén M. (2003). Role of topical emollients and moisturizers in the treatment of dry skin barrier disorders. *American Journal of Clinical Dermatology, 4*(11), 771–788.

17 Ghadially, R., Halkier-Sorensen, L., & Elias, P. M. (1992). Effects of petrolatum on stratum corneum structure and function. *Journal of the American Academy of Dermatology, 26*(3 Pt 2), 387–396.

18 Durai, P. C., Thappa, D. M., Kumari, R., & Malathi, M. (2012). Aging in elderly: Chronological versus photoaging. *Indian Journal of Dermatology, 57*(5), 343–352.

Chapter 6

1   Baker, F. C., Lampio, L., Saaresranta, T., & Polo-Kantola, P. (2018). Sleep and sleep disorders in the menopausal transition. *Sleep Medicine Clinics, 13*(3), 443–456.

2   Bansal, R., & Aggarwal, N. (2019). Menopausal hot flashes: A concise review. *Journal of Mid-Life Health, 10*(1), 6–13.

3   Fisher, W., & Thurston, R. (2016). Measuring hot flash phenomenonology using ambulatory prospective digital diaries. *Menopause, 23*(11), 1222–1227.

4   Archer, D. F., Sturdee, D. W., Baber, R., de Villiers, T. J., Pines, A., Freedman, R. R., Gompel, A., Hickey, M., Hunter, M. S., Lobo, R. A., Lumsden, M. A., MacLennan, A. H., Maki, P., Palacios, S., Shah, D., Villaseca, P., & Warren, M. (2011). Menopausal hot flushes and night sweats: Where are we now? *Climacteric: The Journal of the International Menopause Society, 14*(5), 515–528.

5   Sturdee, D. W., Hunter, M. S., Maki, P. M., Gupta, P., Sassarini, J., Stevenson, J. C., & Lumsden, M. A. (2017). The menopausal hot flush: a review. *Climacteric: the Journal of the International Menopause Society, 20*(4), 296–305.

6   Archer, D. F., Sturdee, D. W., Baber, R., de Villiers, T. J., Pines, A., & Freedman, R. R., Gompel, A., Hickey, M., Hunter, M. S., Lobo, R. A., Lumsden, M. A., MacLennan, A. H., Maki, P., Palacios, S., Shah, D., Villaseca, P., Warren, M. (2011). Menopausal hot flushes and night sweats: where are we now? *Climacteric, 14*(5), 515–528.

7   Stachowiak, G., Pertyński, T., & Pertyńska-Marczewska, M. (2015). Metabolic disorders in menopause. *Przeglad Menopauzalny [Menopause Review], 14*(1), 59–64.

8   Freeman, E. W., Sammel, M. D., & Sanders, R. J. (2014). Risk of long-term hot flashes after natural menopause: Evidence from the Penn Ovarian Aging Study cohort. *Menopause, 21*(9), 924–932.

9   Labrie, F. (2015). All sex steroids are made intracellularly in peripheral tissues by the mechanisms of intracrinology after menopause. *The Journal of Steroid Biochemistry and Molecular Biology, 145*, 133–138.

Chapter 7

1   Labrie, F. (2015). All sex steroids are made intracellularly in peripheral tissues by the mechanisms of intracrinology after menopause. *The Journal of Steroid Biochemistry and Molecular Biology, 145*, 133–138.

2   Martin, K., & Barbieri, R. (2020). Preparations for menopausal hormone therapy. Retrieved from https://www.uptodate.com/contents/preparations-for-menopausal-hormone-therapy

3   Maclennan, A. H., Broadbent, J. L., Lester, S., & Moore, V. (2004). Oral oestrogen and combined oestrogen/progestogen therapy versus placebo for hot flushes. *The Cochrane Database of Systematic Reviews, 4*, CD002978. https://doi.org/10.1002/14651858.CD002978.pub2

4   Keep P.A., Kellerhals J. The ageing woman. In: Lauritzen C., van Keep P.A., editors. Ageing and Estrogens. Frontiers of Hormone Research, Proceedings of the 1st International Workshop on Estrogen Therapy,

Geneva, Switzerland, 1972. Volume 2. S. Karger; Basel, Switzerland: 1973. pp. 160–173.

5   Maclennan, A. H., Broadbent, J. L., Lester, S., & Moore, V. (2004). Oral oestrogen and combined oestrogen/progestogen therapy versus placebo for hot flushes. *Cochrane Database of Systematic Reviews*, *2004*(4), CD002978.

6   Colditz, G. A., Manson, J. E., & Hankinson, S. E. (1997). The Nurses' Health Study: 20-year contribution to the understanding of health among women. *Journal of Women's Health*, *6*(1), 49–62.

7   Million Women Study Collaborative Group (1999). The Million Women Study: design and characteristics of the study population. The Million Women Study Collaborative Group. *Breast Cancer Research*, *1*(1), 73–80.

8   Rossouw, J. E., Anderson, G. L., Prentice, R. L., LaCroix, A. Z., Kooperberg, C., Stefanick, M. L., Jackson, R. D., Beresford, S. A., Howard, B. V., Johnson, K. C., Kotchen, J. M., Ockene, J., & Writing Group for the Women's Health Initiative Investigators (2002). Risks and benefits of estrogen plus progestin in healthy postmenopausal women: principal results From the Women's Health Initiative randomized controlled trial. *Journal of the American Medical Association*, *288*(3), 321–333.

9   Manson, J. E., Chlebowski, R. T., Stefanick, M. L., Aragaki, A. K., Rossouw, J. E., Prentice, R. L., Anderson, G., Howard, B. V., Thomson, C. A., LaCroix, A. Z., Wactawski-Wende, J., Jackson, R. D., Limacher, M., Margolis, K. L., Wassertheil-Smoller, S., Beresford, S. A., Cauley, J. A., Eaton, C. B., Gass, M., Hsia, J., Johnson, K. C., Kooperberg, C., Kuller, L. H., Lewis, C. E., Liu, S., Martin, L. W., Ockene, J. K., O'Sullivan, M. J., Powell, L. H., Simon, M. S., Van Horn, L., Vitolins, M. Z, & Wallace, R. B. (2013). Menopausal hormone therapy and health outcomes during the intervention and extended poststopping phases of the Women's Health Initiative randomized trials. *Journal of the American Medical Association*, *310*(13), 1353–1368.

Chapter 8

1   Cumming, G. P., Currie, H., Morris, E., Moncur, R., & Lee, A. J. (2015). The need to do better – Are we still letting our patients down and at what cost? *Post Reproductive Health*, *21*(2), 56–62.

2   Endocrine Society (2019). Compound Bioidentical Hormone Therapy: An Endocrine Society Position Statement. Retrieved from: https://www.endocrine.org/advocacy/position-statements/compounded-bioidentical-hormone-therapy, accessed 24/01/2021.

3   Mahaguna, V., McDermott, J. M., Zhang, F., & Ochoa, F. (2004). Investigation of product quality between extemporaneously compounded progesterone vaginal suppositories and an approved progesterone vaginal gel. *Drug Development and Industrial Pharmacy*, *30*(10), 1069–1078.

4   Gaudard, A. I. S., Silva de Souza, S., Puga, M. E. S., Marjoribanks, J., da Silva, E. M. K., Torloni, M. R. (2016). Bioidentical hormones for women with vasomotor symptoms. *Cochrane Database of Systematic Reviews, 2016*(8), CD010407.

5   Evans, M. L., Pritts, E., Vittinghoff, E., McClish, K., Morgan, K. S., Jaffe, R. B. (2005). Management of postmenopausal hot flushes with venlafaxine hydrochloride: A randomized, controlled trial. *Obstetric Gynecology, 105*(1), 161-6.

6   Freeman, E. W., Guthrie, K. A., Caan, B., Sternfeld, B., Cohen, L. S., Joffe, H., Carpenter, J. S., Anderson, G. L., Larson, J. C., Ensrud, K. E., Reed, S. D., Newton, K. M., Sherman, S., Sammel, M. D., & LaCroix, A. Z. (2011). Efficacy of escitalopram for hot flashes in healthy menopausal women: A randomized controlled trial. *Journal of the American Medical Association, 305*(3), 267–274.

7   Evans, M. L., Pritts, E., Vittinghoff, E., McClish, K., Morgan, K. S., Jaffe, R. B. (2005). Management of postmenopausal hot flushes with venlafaxine hydrochloride: A randomized, controlled trial. *Obstetric Gynecology, 105*(1), 161-6.

8   Nelson, H. D., Vesco, K. K., Haney, E., Fu, R., Nedrow, A., Miller, J., Nicolaidis, C., Walker, M., & Humphrey, L. (2006). Nonhormonal therapies for menopausal hot flashes: Systematic review and meta-analysis. *Journal of the American Medical Association, 295*(17), 2057–2071.

9   Allameh, Z., Rouholamin, S., & Valaie, S. (2013). Comparison of gabapentin with estrogen for treatment of hot flashes in post-menopausal women. *Journal of Research in Pharmacy Practice, 2*(2), 64–69.

10 National Center for Complementary and Integrative Health. (2018). Complementary, alternative, or integrative health: What's in a Name? Retrieved from: https://www.nccih.nih.gov/health/complementary-alternative-or-integrative-health-whats-in-a-name.

11 Gartoulla, P., Davis, S. R., Worsley, R., & Bell, R. J. (2015). Use of complementary and alternative medicines for menopausal symptoms in Australian women aged 40–65 years. *Medical Journal of Australia, 203*(3), 146–146.

12 Gentry-Maharaj, A., Karpinskyj, C., Glazer, C., Burnell, M. Burnell, Ryan, A., Fraser, L., Lanceley, A., Jacobs, I., Hunter, M. S., & Menon, U. (2015). Use and perceived efficacy of complementary and alternative medicines after discontinuation of hormone therapy: a nested United Kingdom Collaborative Trial of Ovarian Cancer Screening cohort study. *Menopause, 22*(4), 384-390.

13 Johnson, A., Roberts, L., & Elkins, G. (2019). Complementary and alternative medicine for menopause. *Journal of Evidence-Based Integrative Medicine, 24*, 2515690X19829380.

14 Leach, M. J. & Moore, V. (2012). Black cohosh (*Cimicifuga* spp.) for menopausal symptoms. *Cochrane Database of Systematic Reviews, 2012*(9), CD007244.

15 Uebelhack, R., Blohmer, J. U., Graubaum, H. J., Busch, R., Gruenwald, J., Wernecke K. D. (2006). Black cohosh and St. John's wort for climacteric complaints: a randomized trial. *Obstetrics & Gynecology, 107*(2 pt 1), 247-255.

16 Shifren, J. L., Gass, M. L. S., for the NAMS Recommendations for Clinical Care of Midlife Women Working Group. (2014). The North American Menopause Society recommendations for clinical care of midlife women. *Menopause, 21*(10), 1038-1062.

17 Low Dog, T., Powell, K. L., & Weisman, S. M. (2003). Critical evaluation of the safety of *Cimicifuga racemosa* in menopause symptom relief. *Menopause, 10*(4), 299–313.

18 Myers S. P., & Vigar V. (2017). Effects of a standardised extract of Trifolium pratense (Promensil) at a dosage of 80mg in the treatment of menopausal hot flushes: A systematic review and meta-analysis. *Phytomedicine, 24*, 141-147.

19 Tang, G. W. (1994). The climacteric of Chinese factory workers. *Maturitas, 19*(3), 177–182.

20 Nagata, C. (2001). Soy product intake and hot flashes in Japanese women: Results from a community-based prospective study. *American Journal of Epidemiology, 153*(8), 790–793.

21 Chedraui, P., San Miguel, G., & Schwager, G. (2011). The effect of soy-derived isoflavones over hot flushes, menopausal symptoms and mood in climacteric women with increased body mass index. *Gynecological Endocrinology, 27*(5), 307–313.

22 Maclennan, A. H., Broadbent, J. L., Lester, S., & Moore, V. (2004). Oral oestrogen and combined oestrogen/progestogen therapy versus placebo for hot flushes. *Cochrane Database of Systematic Reviews, 2004*(4), CD002978.

23 Carmignani, L. O., Pedro, A. O., Costa-Paiva, L. H., & Pinto-Neto, A. M. (2010). The effect of dietary soy supplementation compared to estrogen and placebo on menopausal symptoms: a randomized controlled trial. *Maturitas, 67*(3), 262–269.

24 Chen, M., Lin, C., & Liu, C. (2014). Efficacy of phytoestrogens for menopausal symptoms: a meta-analysis and systematic review. *Climacteric, 18*(2), 260–269.

25 Hill-Sakurai, L. E., Muller, J., & Thom, D. H. (2008). Complementary and alternative medicine for menopause: a qualitative analysis of women's decision making. *Journal of General Internal Medicine, 23*(5), 619–622.

26 Endocrine Society (2019). Compound Bioidentical Hormone Therapy: An Endocrine Society Position Statement. Retrieved from: https://

www.endocrine.org/advocacy/position-statements/compounded-bioidentical-hormone-therapy, accessed 24/01/2021.

27 Gaudard, A. I. S., Silva de Souza, S., Puga, M. E. S., Marjoribanks, J., da Silva, E. M. K., Torloni, M. R. (2016). Bioidentical hormones for women with vasomotor symptoms. *Cochrane Database of Systematic Reviews, 2016*(8), CD010407.

Chapter 9

1 Kravitz, H. M., & Joffe, H. (2011). Sleep during the perimenopause: a SWAN story. *Obstetrics and Gynecology Clinics of North America, 38*(3), 567–586.

2 Eugene, A. R., Masiak, J. (2015). The neuroprotective aspects of sleep. *MEDtube Science, 3*(1), 35-40.

3 Buysse, D. J., Angst, J., Gamma, A., Ajdacic, V., Eich, D., & Rössler, W. (2008). Prevalence, course, and comorbidity of insomnia and depression in young adults. *Sleep, 31*(4), 473–480.

4 NIH State-of-the-Science Conference Statement on Management of Menopause-Related Symptoms. (2005, March 21–32). *NIH Consensus and State-of-the-Science Statements, 22*(1) 1–38.

5 Kravitz, H., & Joffe, H. (2011). Sleep during the perimenopause: A SWAN story. *Obstetrics and Gynecology Clinics of North America, 38*(3), 567–586.

6 Freedman, R. R., & Roehrs, T. A. (2006). Effects of REM sleep and ambient temperature on hot flash-induced sleep disturbance. *Menopause, 13*(4), 576–583.

7 Miller, E. H. (2004). Women and insomnia. *Clinical cornerstone, 6 Suppl 1B*, S8–S18.

8 Dennerstein, L., Lehert, P., Burger, H. G., & Guthrie, J. R. (2007). New findings from non-linear longitudinal modelling of menopausal hormone changes. *Human Reproduction Update, 13*(6), 551–557.

9 Kalleinen, N., Polo-Kantola, P., Irjala, K., Porkka-Heiskanen, T., Vahlberg, T., Virkki, A., & Polo, O. (2008). 24-hour serum levels of growth hormone, prolactin, and cortisol in pre- and postmenopausal women: the effect of combined estrogen and progestin treatment. *The Journal of Clinical Endocrinology and Metabolism, 93*(5), 1655–1661.

10 Gottesmann C. (2002). GABA mechanisms and sleep. *Neuroscience, 111*(2), 231–239.

11 Prather, A., Puterman, E., Epel, E., & Dhabhar, F. (2014). Poor sleep quality potentiates stress-induced cytokine reactivity in postmenopausal women with high visceral abdominal adiposity. *Brain, Behavior, and Immunity, 35*, 155–162.

12 Gallicchio, L., & Kalesan, B. (2009). Sleep duration and mortality: a systematic review and meta-analysis. *Journal of Sleep Research, 18*(2), 148–158.

13   Moreno-Frías, C., Figueroa-Vega, N., & Malacara, J. M. (2014). Relationship of sleep alterations with perimenopausal and postmenopausal symptoms. *Menopause, 21*(9), 1017–1022.

14   Leach, M. J., & Page, A. T. (2015). Herbal medicine for insomnia: A systematic review and meta-analysis. *Sleep Medicine Reviews, 24,* 1–12.

15   Taslaman, M. (2014). The efficacy and safety of herbal medicine for insomnia in adults: An overview of recent research. *Australian Journal of Herbal Medicine, 26*(3), 86-93.

16   Reddy, S., Reddy, V., & Sharma, S. (2020). *Physiology, Circadian Rhythm* [Ebook]. Treasure Island (FL): StatPearls [Internet]. Retrieved from https://www.ncbi.nlm.nih.gov/books/NBK519507/

17   Tähkämö, L., Partonen, T., & Pesonen, A. K. (2019). Systematic review of light exposure impact on human circadian rhythm. *Chronobiology International, 36*(2), 151–170.

18   Dodson, E. R., & Zee, P. C. (2010). Therapeutics for Circadian Rhythm Sleep Disorders. *Sleep Medicine Clinics, 5*(4), 701–715.

19   Sivertsen, B., Omvik, S., Pallesen, S., Bjorvatn, B., Havik, O. E., Kvale, G., Nielsen, G. H., & Nordhus, I. H. (2006). Cognitive behavioral therapy vs zopiclone for treatment of chronic primary insomnia in older adults: A randomized controlled trial. *Journal of the American Medical Association, 295*(24), 2851-2858.

20   McCurry, S. M., Guthrie, K. A., Morin, C. M., Woods, N. F., Landis, C. A., Ensrud, K. E., Larson, J. C., Joffe, H., Cohen, L. S., Hunt, J. R., Newton, K. M., Otte, J. L., Reed, S. D., Sternfeld, B., Tinker, L. F., & LaCroix, A. Z. (2016). Telephone-based cognitive behavioral therapy for insomnia in perimenopausal and postmenopausal women with vasomotor symptoms: A MsFLASH randomized clinical trial. *Journal of the American Medical Association Internal Medicine, 176*(7), 913–920.

21   Ye, Y. Y., Chen, N. K., Chen, J., Liu, J., Lin, L., Liu, Y. Z., Lang, Y., Li, X. J., Yang, X. J., & Jiang, X. J. (2016). Internet-based cognitive-behavioural therapy for insomnia (ICBT-i): A meta-analysis of randomised controlled trials. *BMJ Open, 6*(11), e010707.

22   Vakkuri, O., Kivelä, A., Leppäluoto, J., Valtonen, M., & Kauppila, A. (1996). Decrease in melatonin precedes follicle-stimulating hormone increase during perimenopause. *European Journal of Endocrinology, 135*(2), 188–192.

23   Zhou, J. N., Liu, R. Y., van Heerikhuize, J., Hofman, M. A., & Swaab, D. F. (2003). Alterations in the circadian rhythm of salivary melatonin begin during middle-age. *Journal of Pineal Research, 34*(1), 11–16.

24   Dodson, E. R., & Zee, P. C. (2010). Therapeutics for circadian rhythm sleep disorders. *Sleep Medicine Clinics, 5*(4), 701–715.

Chapter 10

1   Dennerstein, L., Alexander, J. L., & Kotz, K. (2003). The menopause and sexual functioning: A review of the population-based studies. *Annual Review of Sex Research, 14*, 64–82.

2   Lavoisier, P., Aloui, R., Schmidt, M. H., & Watrelot, A. (1995). Clitoral blood flow increases following vaginal pressure stimulation. *Archives of Sexual Behavior, 24*(1), 37–45.

3   Inayat, K., Danish, N., & Hassan, L. (2017). Symptoms of menopause in peri and postmenopausal women and their attitude towards them. *Journal of Ayub Medical College, Abbottabad, 29*(3), 477–480.

4   Avis, N. E., Brockwell, S., Randolph, J. F., Jr, Shen, S., Cain, V. S., Ory, M., & Greendale, G. A. (2009). Longitudinal changes in sexual functioning as women transition through menopause: Results from the Study of Women's Health Across the Nation. *Menopause, 16*(3), 442–452.

5   Davis, S., & Jane, F. (2011). *Sex and perimenopause* [Ebook]. Royal Australian College of General Practitioners. Retrieved from https://www.racgp.org.au/download/documents/AFP/2011/May/201105davis.pdf

6   Biehl, C., Plotsker, O., & Mirkin, S. (2019). A systematic review of the efficacy and safety of vaginal estrogen products for the treatment of genitourinary syndrome of menopause. *Menopause, 26*(4), 431–453.

7   Franco, O. H., Chowdhury, R., Troup, J., Voortman, T., Kunutsor, S., Kavousi, M., Oliver-Williams, C., & Muka, T. (2016). Use of Plant-Based Therapies and Menopausal Symptoms: A Systematic Review and Meta-analysis. *Journal of the American Medical Association, 315*(23), 2554–2563.

Chapter 12

1   Jones, H. J., Huang, A. J., Subak, L. L., Brown, J. S., & Lee, K. A. (2016). Bladder symptoms in the early menopausal transition. *Journal of Women's Health (2002), 25*(5), 457–463. https://doi.org/10.1089/jwh.2015.5370.

2   Dumoulin C., Cacciari L. P., Hay⊠Smith E. J. C. (2008) Pelvic floor muscle training versus no treatment, or inactive control treatments, for urinary incontinence in women. *Cochrane Database of Systematic Reviews, 10*, CD005654.

3   Department of Health. (2018). *National Women's Health Strategy 2020-2030*. Canberra: Commonwealth of Australia. Retrieved from https://www1.health.gov.au/internet/main/publishing.nsf/Content/AF504671BA9786E8CA2583D6000AFAE7/$File/National%20Womens%20Health%20Strategy%202020-2030.pdf

4   Kidney Health Australia (2020). What is kidney disease? Retrieved from https://kidney.org.au/your-kidneys/what-is-kidney-disease

5   Abelson, B., Sun, D., Que, L., Nebel, R. A., Baker, D., Popiel, P., Amundsen, C. L., Chai, T., Close, C., DiSanto, M., Fraser, M. O., Kielb, S. J., Kuchel, G., Mueller, E. R., Palmer, M. H., Parker-Autry, C., Wolfe, A. J., & Damaser, M. S. (2018). Sex differences in lower urinary tract biology and physiology. *Biology of Sex Differences, 9*(1), 45.

6   Fu, Z., Liska, D., Talan, D., & Chung, M. (2017). Cranberry reduces the risk of urinary tract infection recurrence in otherwise healthy women: A systematic review and meta-analysis. *The Journal of Nutrition, 147*(12), 2282–2288.

7   Shao, Y., Forster, S. C., Tsaliki, E., Vervier, K., Strang, A., Simpson, N., Kumar, N., Stares, M. D., Rodger, A., Brocklehurst, P., Field, N., & Lawley, T. D. (2019). Stunted microbiota and opportunistic pathogen colonization in caesarean-section birth. *Nature, 574*(7776), 117–121.